The

Modern Yoga
Bible

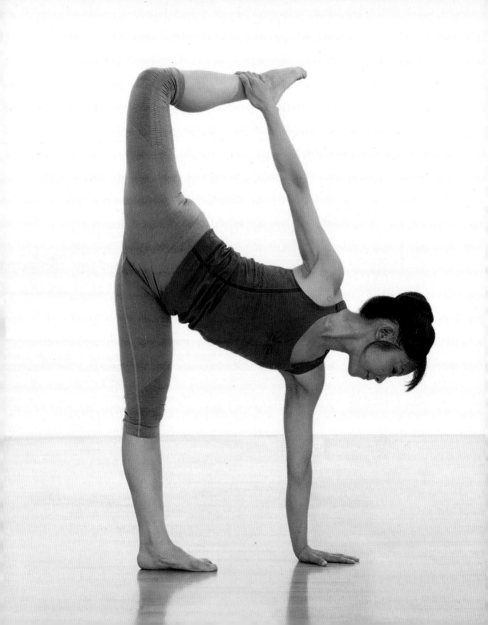

The
Modern Yoga
Bible

Christina Brown

The definitive guide to yoga today

WALKING
STICK
PRESS

Published in the U.S. by Walking Stick Press, an imprint of F+W Media, Inc.
10151 Carver Road, Suite #200, Blue Ash, OH 45242
(800) 289-0963

First published in Great Britain in 2015 by Godsfield Press,
a division of Octopus Publishing Group Ltd, Carmelite House,
50 Victoria Embankment
London EC4Y 0DZ

www.octopusbooks.co.uk

Disclaimer
The author and publisher disclaim to any person or entity, any liability, loss,
or damage caused or alleged to be caused, directly or indirectly as a result
of the use, application, or interpretation of any of the contents of this book.
All information and/or advice given in this book should not take the place
of any medical, counselling, legal, or financial advice given to you by any
qualified professional.

Christina Brown asserts the moral right to be identified as the author of
this work.

ISBN: 978-1-4403-4555-5

A CIP catalogue record for this book is available from the British Library.

Printed and bound in China.

10 9 8 7 6 5 4 3 2 1

Commissioning Editor: Leanne Bryan
Art Director: Yasia Williams-Leedham
Senior Editor: Alex Stetter
Designer: Sally Bond
Special Photography: Ruth Jenkinson, Colin Husband
Production Controller: Allison Gonsalves

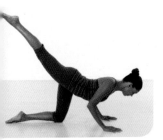
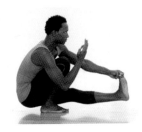
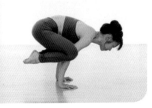
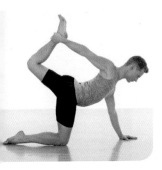

contents

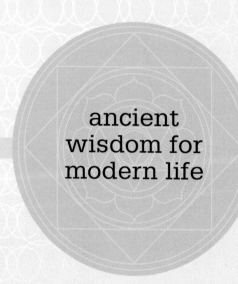

ancient wisdom for modern life

ATHA अथ

The *Yoga Sutras*, as a codification of Hatha yoga, is an important classic text, containing 196 concise aphorisms that tell us exactly what steps to take to achieve the goals of Hatha yoga. The first line of the *Yoga Sutras* – *atha yoganusasanam* – means: "Now, the teaching of yoga". So *atha* is the very first word of the very first line of the Sutras. While it's meant as an introduction to the remaining instructions, to me it means something more. What I love about it is that if you can *truly* understand and integrate this first word – *now* – you actually may not need the rest. If you can fully apply the concept of bringing your mind to the present moment, then you will be free. It's liberating to allow the past to drop away and to let the fantasies of the future have less of an imprint. When you exist in the

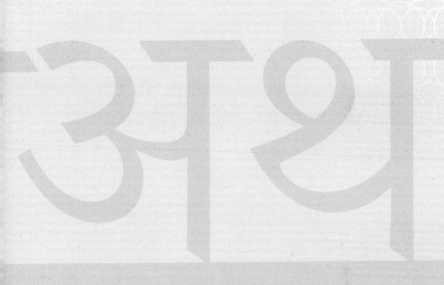

present moment, so much stress just falls away. It is a beautiful experience to be present to life as it unfolds.

Try chanting it: "*Aa-Tha*" – the *h* gives the second syllable a slight aspirated sound. The first syllable is a slightly longer sound, with a rising intonation, and the second is a shorter, falling intonation.

> *If you can fully apply the concept of bringing your mind to the present moment, then you will be free.*

Part 1

INTRODUCTION

The Benefits of Yoga

Do you know why you have opened this book? Yoga meets so many needs, it's no wonder its popularity has grown and grown. While you may come to yoga with a physiotherapeutic goal in mind – hoping to ease body aches and pains – it probably won't take you too many yoga classes to discover some of the other benefits. For many, yoga develops into something that is more than just about lengthening and strengthening. It becomes about living life better outside the yoga room.

I am guessing that you could be looking at this book because you would like to feel calmer, more peaceful and a little happier. To me, what's most beautiful about yoga practice is how expanded and spacious I feel, both during and after it. When you find a practice that suits you well, it's easy to get into a flow-zone that

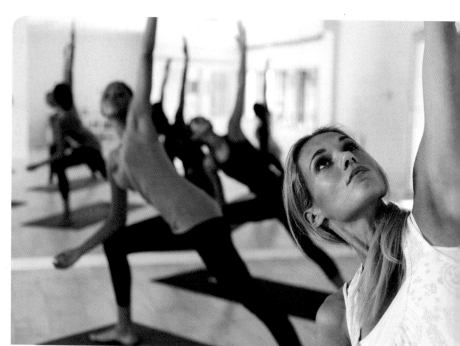

is very uplifting, and this can resonate long afterward. One of my students explained how he often felt after class: "It's as if all is right with the world." This is not insignificant. In a world where the daily news features tragic stories of war, disaster, misfortune and violence, it can feel as if there is frequently little that is positive out there for us. We need to be able to peep our heads above any clouds of anger and hate that hang over us. Yoga provides essential relief to the darker elements of our worldscape. It reminds us that we can rise above aggression and hatred and live well.

Yoga practice allows me to re-experience the beauty of who I am, and to experience my body as a sanctuary. In a world where we are often encouraged to be busy and materially productive, spending time on yourself can be seen as selfish. I often remind my students how, when you love someone very much, it is natural to want to spend time with them. It becomes simple and effortless to give that person your time. Rolling out your mat ready for practice is an affirmation that you want to devote time to yourself. It is a great act of love toward yourself and, from that, it becomes deeply healing. The bottom line is that you can be happier practising yoga. And you deserve to feel this way.

LEFT: *A regular yoga practice can make you feel calm and peaceful, as well as more limber.*

Yoga: science or spirituality?

When you follow the guidelines from the ancient texts, yoga is a science. It offers us a logical series of steps that help us to live better. The aim of yoga is to clear the mind, improve the quality of the mind and understand the reality of the mind. The active postures, or *asanas*, that make up most of this book are a helping hand to the purpose of yoga. They will keep your body healthy, strong and limber. They also prepare the body to sit with ease, so that you can practise the mental focusing techniques that will help clear your mind. This is all a terrific antidote to whichever imbalances are occurring in your day-to-day life. As you read on, you will find that yoga has a solid basis. But yoga is also an art and, with that, a little bit mysterious and magical. How else can simply making a series of shapes with our bodies have such a profound effect on our psyche, make us feel so incredibly good and create such a vast number of yoga enthusiasts worldwide?

Unlike Western psychology, which has tended to focus on understanding those who are sick, Eastern psychology long ago figured out the importance of positive thinking. Two thousand years ago, Eastern yogis (practitioners of yoga) had already completed an in-depth study of the nature of *healthy* minds, worked out how to achieve self-realization and outlined how to deal with the pitfalls encountered en route. Their techniques are sound and time-tested. And what they discovered holds truer than ever today. While our modern lives arguably see us moving ever further from our roots and from that which keeps us grounded, those wise old yogis are still holding a beacon of light and truth, to guide the rest of us forward.

In this book there are references to the two most-discussed ancient texts: the *Hatha Yoga Pradipika* and the *Yoga Sutras*. The *Hatha Yoga Pradipika* was written in the 15th century CE by Svātmārāma; the important source known as the *Yoga Sutras* (see also pages 6 and 14–16) is a collection of aphorisms codified by the sage Patanjali in about 400 CE. The *Yoga Sutras* are like a recipe book, describing step-by-step what we need to do to achieve *Kaivalyam*, the ultimate freedom. You'll find quotes and inspiration from the *Sutras* throughout the book, to guide you in your approach to modern life.

Yoga postures and breathing

This book is about Hatha yoga, which is one of several branches of yoga. It is the "yoga of effort" – the active yoga exercises most commonly practised around the world today. Yoga was originally taught by oral transmission in Sanskrit, the language used by scholars. *Asana* is the Sanskrit word for the physical postures that are familiar to yoga practitioners worldwide. The literal definition of *asana* is "seat", because you either "sit" into a yoga shape or are comfortably seated to be able to move and take action in the world with ease. The *asanas* are one of the "limbs" of yoga, and there are seven others. Another limb encompasses the breathing techniques (*pranayama*).

Ethical codes of conduct

Other limbs of Hatha yoga relate to its profound and ancient philosophy, which amazingly covers everything you need to do to be able to achieve an enlightened state. You can read more about the philosophy in the "Ancient wisdom for modern life" sections that you'll find dotted throughout this book.

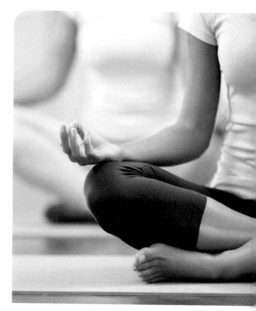

Hatha yoga also includes two limbs that cover the ethical principles of living, and these are called the *yama* and *niyama*. Together they form a list of ten ethical observances that protect and support healthy relational boundaries with yourself and others.

The five *yamas* encompass your intentions, thoughts and actions. They are ancient concepts, and yet they still offer modern people a perfect set of guidelines for living. They are:

- *Ahimsa* – holding an intention of doing no harm to others
- *Satya* – speaking truthfully
- *Asteya* – not taking what does not belong to you, or that which is not willingly given
- *Brahmacharya* – conserving your energy for your highest aspiration
- *Aparigraha* – taking only what is sufficient for your needs to support you in living in alignment with your environment and the people with whom you are in contact.

The five *niyamas* incorporate discipline in actions and attitudes toward yourself. Although they were also written more than two thousand years ago, these principles are as relevant today as they were then. Put simply, it's easier to be gentle toward, and respect, others if you follow these guidelines:

- *Saucha* – take care of yourself
- *Santosha* – enjoy what you have in your life
- *Tapas* – apply some discipline to achieve your goals
- *Swadhyaya* – understand yourself deeply through self-study
- *Ishvarapranidhana* – recognize that ultimately you are not wholly responsible for the way things turn out, and that the world is greater than you.

Focus, concentration, meditation and enlightenment

You may already associate the next three limbs with yoga practice. A certain withdrawal of the senses (*pratyahara*, the fifth limb) is useful. It's more challenging to have a quiet mind with a loud lifestyle; it's harder to have a focused mind with an action-filled life. Toning down the constant stimulation of the senses will leave you better positioned to develop your concentration (*dharana*, the sixth limb), in order to be able to achieve a deeply meditative mental state (*dhyana*, the seventh limb).

The eighth and final limb – and the aim of Hatha yoga – is *samadhi*, which can be translated as "bliss". It's an experience that will occur as a result of the seven other limbs. This natural state of being, the *samadhi* state, is an experience of oneness.

LEFT: *The Sanskrit word for the physical yoga postures,* asana, *literally means "seat".*

Modern yoga – a great workout and a superb work-*in*

The essence of yoga is outlined in the first four points of Patanjali's *Yoga Sutras*:

1. The purpose of yoga is outlined in the first *sutra*, written in Sanskrit as *Yogash citta vritti nirodhah*. This tells us that the state of yoga is the cessation of the movements of the mind.

2. The second *sutra* informs us that the mind is the tool, and the way to quiet the mind is to work *with* the mind. Only with a clean, clear mind can we be in touch with the truth of the moment.

3. The third *sutra* tells us that the mind is also the goal. When we are in the state of yoga, we won't be led astray by distorted understanding or incorrect thoughts. This *sutra* informs us that there is no aspect of our lives that is untouched when we perceive things in their true nature. It shines a different light on everything. Once we can better understand reality, we can be helped to avoid the causes of pain and will have control over more than we may imagine.

4. The fourth *sutra* tells us that the mind is actually also part of the problem. This is because when the mind is disturbed, it is unable to follow a direction or to comprehend things accurately. In this case, we will move away from the state of yoga.

The remaining 192 *sutras* are an elaboration of these first four. If you want to experience peace within, the *Yoga Sutras* will take you through the steps that will lead you toward quieting the mind and existing in the peaceful state of yoga.

From the *Yoga Sutras* we learn that only when we are in the state of yoga will we know things as they truly are. When the mind is not in that state, we are unable to see the true nature of things. So the aim of yoga practice is to achieve a sustained mental quietness, in order to be fully present and therefore able to understand and reflect true nature. It's a lofty goal, isn't it? So I understand if you simply want to focus on stretching out those tight hamstrings, for the time being. But hang around yoga classes for long enough and your curiosity may develop further, as those quiet relaxations at the end of the session offer you more than just a glimmer of a new, very peaceful way of being.

Breathe through a sudden surge of emotion that arises unexpectedly in a forward bend, and feel yourself transformed and somehow uplifted. As you exit the yoga room, you might feel like a nicer, calmer, kinder or more tolerant person. Or perhaps, when you are deeply touched by some event in your life, you may find yourself guided through the doorway of yoga into discovering your inner world. And you may find that your inner world is a sanctuary. Your *asana* practice is then elevated beyond being simply a physical workout or an effective de-stressing tool. As your body, mind and psyche are inevitably intertwined, your Hatha yoga practice may become a soothing place of solace for the heart, and a rewarding journey of self-development.

Why modern yoga?

Hatha yoga practice has evolved considerably since my original book, *The Yoga Bible* (now available as *The Classic Yoga Bible*), was written 15 years ago. Thanks to advances in movement sciences and more in-depth training, the therapeutic side of the physical postures has developed. The popularity of Pilates means that modern yoga puts greater emphasis on strength and careful alignment in the pelvis, shoulder, back and abdomen. For example, modern yoga classes now often feature a whole range of core-strengthening practices that are quite different from what was on offer a decade and a half ago.

Happily, yoga has moved from hippy to mainstream, and en route it has opened up to more influences. Any art practised more widely is bound to be influenced by the previous training of its practitioners. Yoga teachers with backgrounds in martial arts, tai chi and qi gong have married some of those principles to

their yoga teachings, as have teachers with other backgrounds: Feldenkrais, the Franklin Method and the Alexander Technique, to name but a few.

In the 1980s yoga was heavily influenced by B K S Iyengar, an accomplished Hatha yogi who is credited with bringing yoga to the West in the 1960s. Iyengar yoga is characterized by long, strong holds that build stamina and flexibility. And throughout the 1990s the popularity of Astanga Vinyasa yoga brought the concept of continued flow into regular yoga practices, spawning other faster, flow-based practices that are popular in the West today.

Some practices feature one movement on each inhalation and another on each exhalation. In other forms, a yoga practitioner might pause for several breaths in a pose, then move straight on to another pose. Flow yoga, in which the movements mirror the breath, is a beautiful adjunct to static poses, where for newer yoga practitioners the breathing can become a little difficult. And so sequencing has become more sophisticated and creative, which means that a yoga practice can feel like a poetic stream of movement.

Thanks to technology, it feels as if life moves faster now than it did 15 years ago. It's as if our attention spans have diminished. So while our interest in flow-yoga practices may reflect how we have sped ourselves up, at the same time there has been a rebound toward a new breed of slow yoga styles. As if to intuitively counterbalance ourselves, restorative yoga and yin yoga have become more important. Restorative yoga features soft, relaxed postures, each held for many minutes; these poses are usually supported with props, to soften the intensity of the poses. Yin yoga borrows from the East, using the meridian (or energy-channel) systems found in Chinese medicine. Rather than trying to change the muscles, it targets the joints and connective tissues; it also features long holds, where the intensity levels can be high in order to strengthen the bones and ligaments.

While it may appear superficially that all these variations of yoga practice provide different choices, in essence yoga remains unchanged, and the original yogic ethos remains eternal. Despite all the changes humankind has been able to manifest over the centuries, and despite the myriad forms of yoga that will continue to evolve, essentially we are still human beings for whom the timeless practices of yoga remain absolutely relevant. The ancient yogis had a fantastic understanding of the mind and how to calm it, and of how to use yoga to care for our inner worlds (ourselves) and our outer worlds (our relationships, other beings and the environment).

Yoga is a practice of evolution. One of the classic definitions of yoga is: to achieve something not able to be reached before. This inevitably results in personal growth and transformation. Aside from the changes in Western yoga in recent decades, anyone who has practised for many years will inevitably evolve themselves. Their needs will alter and, as they do, their yoga practice will naturally tend to change. Longtime yogis may relate to my own journey, which began as a teenager in some sort of search for physical perfection – and with a healthy dose of ego. Over the years it has changed from a more cerebral search to understand each pose to the nth degree, accompanied by attempts to attain "perfect" alignment or to achieve the hardest possible variation of a pose, to become one that is much less demanding and more of a reliable long-term relationship. I now have a much softer attitude, a softer practice and, with that, a delightful sense of fun and play. Thankfully I rarely feel the pressure of having to "prove" anything. My relationship with yoga has evolved into a nurturing, stable and rewarding marriage, and it serves me well.

RIGHT: *Restorative and yin yoga feature soft postures that are held for longer periods of time.*

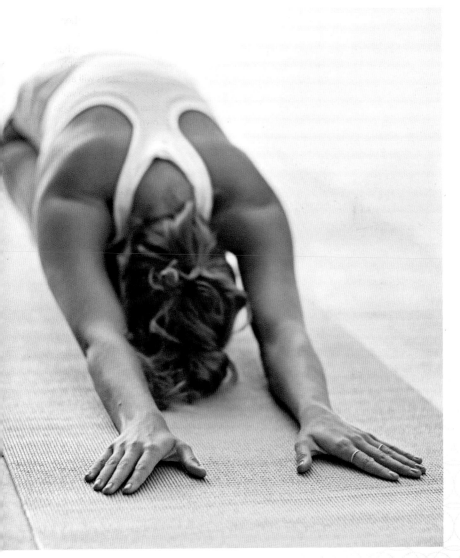

How yoga makes you feel so good

Yoga and positive psychology – the state of flow

In positive psychology the concept of "flow-states" has become popular, thanks to research by the Hungarian psychologist Mihaly Csikszentmihalyi and his colleagues. The flow-state is an experience of deep focus and rapture while you are performing an activity. This experience, when you have full involvement and enjoyment of the activity, is also known as being "in the zone". It's a pleasurable state in which you feel complete absorption and where time flies. You can experience flow in many places: during study, at work, while playing music, making love, playing sport and during yoga practice.

Yoga scores highly in "flow" rankings when compared to other sports activities in general. Ideally, during your Hatha yoga practice, there is a loss of self-consciousness as your ego-state softens and you lose your fear of failure. To make it more likely to reach the state of flow, you need to balance your abilities with your attitude and the level of difficulty of your postures. If you are choosing a simple practice that is very easy for you, it's even more important to approach each pose in a curious, thorough and mindful way. When you approach a familiar pose as if it's your first time, we call it "the beginner's mind". The freshness of the beginner's mind will increase the likelihood of you opening to the state of flow. Otherwise, apathy or boredom will move you away from the flow experience. As your skill in the postures increases, so too can the challenge of the postures that you choose. With skill and challenge nicely balanced, you lay the foundations for an optimal experience of flow. If the challenge of the postures is too high for your skill level, anxiety will result. And, as you will have gathered by now, anxiety is not the aim of Hatha yoga practice, but rather the opposite.

Yoga and neuroplasticity

When my original *Yoga Bible* was written 15 years ago, it was thought that the brain was hard-wired by the age of five or six, but we have now updated our understanding of the concept of neuroplasticity – the brain's ability to reorganize itself. Neuroplasticity has shown that our brains are in a constant state of reorganization, depending on how they are being used. Repeated, consistent patterns created by new experiences can change the brain. (You can think of the brain as a bit like a muscle: the worked-out bits get stronger, while the unused parts get weaker.) With this in mind, it becomes important to fortify positive patterns, and the yoga texts were all clear on this millennia ago. They stressed the importance of a consistent yoga practice as the key to success. Consistent practice affects how we feel, how we deal with our emotions, how aware we are of our bodies and how integrated we are on all levels. These benefits carry through to life off the yoga mat.

Neuroplasticity also tells us what happens when we connect our intention and concentration with our breath and physical movement. Over time we form a positive association and it feels good. There's even a catchphrase for how the neural pathways behave: "What fires together, wires together." This is why you can quickly "drop in" to your pleasant "yoga zone" as soon as you stand on your yoga mat. You may notice that the first single upward sweep with your arms in a Sun Salute makes you instantly feel better, more harmoniously integrated, calm and at ease. It also means that, after some time with a regular meditation practice, you can centre yourself down to a deep, meditative mindset fairly efficiently when you sit.

It's important to realize that the continued rewiring of the brain works the other way, too. Each time you feel stressed, you are reinforcing the neural networks for that uncomfortable experience. This is where regularity of practice is important, so that you can continue to amplify the good stuff and dampen down whatever you don't want to reinforce.

The nervous system has a neat reward system, of which Hatha yoga is perfectly positioned to take full advantage. The body releases feel-good chemicals called dopamine and endorphins. While there are lots of other experiences that can make this happen as well – listening to music, communal experience and other types of exercise – there is a kind of sacred biochemistry with Hatha yoga practice. During yoga the combination of mindfulness, deep breathing and movement triggers the release of these chemicals, amplifying the positive rewiring of the brain, and transformation occurs.

A good thing to add to this mix is the Loving-Kindness Meditation (see page 372), which will help you to develop compassion and feel beautifully connected to the community around you. And do practise the Mindfulness Meditations and Gratitude (see pages 366 and 370) before or after your active yoga practices. Mindfulness, deep breathing and slowing movement plus meditation are the perfect ingredients to help you become less reactive, heal old wounds and deal with stress better. You will become more appreciative of all you are and have. You will feel happier and healthier, enjoy your body more, open more fully to love and feel more at peace in the world.

How to use this book

In this book you will touch and taste elements of the concepts mentioned above. You will find yoga practices to suit your own needs. There are practices for each different day and decade, as your ability, energy levels and moods naturally change. There are postures to make you strong and supple, and ones to freshen and refocus your mind. There are practices to calm your emotions and make your heart sing; there are experiences of serenity for your soul, as you touch that nugget of peace that always resides within you, although sometimes you're just too busy to notice it.

To create the greatest impact in a short amount of time, there are lots of combination poses, where the leg position of one classic pose is matched with, say, the shoulder-stretching arm action of another. There are also many flowing postures, which can reduce the intensity and keep your breathing steady, so that you'll feel good while you practise. I have added a healthy dose of longer holds and lots of emphasis on alignment; and I recommend doing a liberal amount of Ocean Breath (see page 332) to keep you focused. Add a sprinkle of meditation and relaxation, some guidance on mindfulness and *voilà* – you have the great workout, with the superb work-*in* that is modern yoga.

To help piece your practice together, follow the sequences outlined on pages 376–87. Alternatively, you can start at the front of the book and choose one or two practices from each section, for a fairly balanced routine. The text boxes include additional suggestions for your practice, so that you can take different journeys on different days; in these boxes you will find the following topics that will help your travels through the book:

- **build up** – offers a suggested preparatory pose
- **move forward** – gives an idea of where to go next in the book; most of these progressions will deepen your practice by continuing on the same theme (for example, moving from an initial twist to a stronger twisting action)
- **balance out** – gives directions to a posture that counterposes the work just done (for example, moving from a twist to a symmetrical pose, such as a forward bend, to help balance you out)
- **unwind** – suggests options to take the intensity down a notch, to an easier or more relaxing posture
- **take care** – indicates that some postures are contraindicated for certain conditions.

One, two, three stars ☆☆☆

Be guided by the star system for the level of challenge. A pose marked with one star is manageable for most bodies;

three stars you might have to build up to. The star rating assumes that you have no injuries or particular restrictions. If you have a current or chronic injury, or any significant tendencies toward certain issues, you will need to adjust poses as necessary. Do refer to each section introduction for general "cautions", and to each pose for any specific contraindications; and be sensible about not pushing yourself to the point of injury, seeking further guidance where necessary. If you have any recent or chronic injury anywhere, work under the supervision of an experienced and knowledgeable teacher.

Be smart and leave your ego off the mat. Don't push into pain, and do seek qualified advice as you need it. Each individual will find that they are looser or weaker in some areas, and tighter or stronger in others. Just because you can achieve an admirable-looking pose that has three stars next to it, don't assume that opens the way for all the other three-star poses. Yoga poses tend to be multifaceted, and they work with many different lines of stretch and areas to strengthen.

Some practices will push your boundaries, requiring courage and acting as a mirror to encourage you to expand the fixed edges in your "real life" off the mat. Other practices are soft, sensual and slinky – the psychological equivalent of sinking into a deep, soothing bath at the end of a long day.

The essence of yoga is timeless, yet in modern times we need it more than ever, as many of our lives fluctuate between stressed-and-wired and stressed-and-tired. Its essence is noble, authentic and deep, but you can still be playful, joyful and open to fun with yoga. I hope you have lots of fun with this book.

Guidelines to practice

- **Just do the best you can.** Applying your best effort each day is much better than achieving a "perfect practice". Your yoga postures don't need to be glamorous or crowd-pleasing. Simple is often best. Neuroplasticity means that mindful practice of simple poses will create new positive patterns of being, and your inner journey is just as important as creating new patterns in your physicality. Progression is, of course, fine as you develop your physical practice, but don't be led astray by the wantings of your ego.

- **Discipline is essential.** You will get results if you practise regularly with dedication, curiosity and enthusiasm. Keep up your enthusiasm by making sure that you choose lots of postures you enjoy doing. Then you will feel good and are more likely to practise. Keep an open mind and explore the things that challenge you, too.

- **Let go of the idea of the perfect pose.** Aim to be perfectly in the moment while you are in any pose.

- **Take breaks during your practice.** This offers you time to learn to access the "in-between" spaces. Your body can then integrate the positive changes, and that's when deep healing occurs.

- **Sthira sukham asanam** (*Yoga Sutras* II:46) is an important *sutra*. It tells us that a yoga pose should be steady and comfortable. You need to remain alert, yet feel relaxed in the postures. A posture shouldn't create burnout and needs to be sustainable. Watch your breath, and change what you are doing if your breath becomes irregular. While each Hatha yoga pose will imprint on the breath, it mustn't stop the flow or make it feel jagged or jarring. Check in with your breathing often. It's the barometer to the way you are feeling.

- **Don't just do something – sit there!** The active practice of the yoga poses by themselves is not enough. You need to explore the breathwork, relaxations and meditations as well. Even five minutes of Mindfulness Meditation (see page 366) can be life-changing if practised daily.

- **Sense, feel and act appropriately** – always with presence and compassion. Every yoga pose offers you the choice of how much effort to put in and how relaxed to be in the pose. More relaxation often means more enjoyment. If you have a rather driven personality, give yourself full permission to hang back from your edge. It may confront you to take things easy, but sometimes the best development means getting out of your comfort zone. The timings offered in this book are guidelines only, so you can set your own thresholds during your practice, in terms of the length of holds and the depth of your movements.

- **Learn to trust your own perceptions.** Use your yoga practice to develop your intuitive skills. Every day you have a whole lot of different cells that you didn't have yesterday. Effectively you have a new body, so meet each pose and each practice afresh.

- **Your identity or value as a person** is not linked to how "perfect" your Lotus pose is, how long you can hold a Headstand or how handsome you appear in a pose. Trust me – at your funeral, nobody will be talking about how long your hamstrings were.

BELOW: *Every yoga pose offers options, letting you choose the version that feels right for you.*

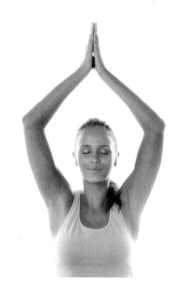

My love-letter to yoga

I am frequently struck with a sense of honour when a student who is brand-new to yoga turns up to class. In the back of my mind is the thought that, for this person, the experience may be the beginning of a lifelong love affair with yoga practices.

Regardless of your experience – brand-new or accomplished yogi – you can delight in your yoga practice. We are all subject to the ups and downs of life, so this doesn't mean your life will always be pain-free. We all have days when our bodies feel stiff, weak or wooden, so it doesn't mean you will feel strong or flexible in every single pose. We all have times when our minds are scattered or lethargic, so it doesn't mean each practice will feel anchored and easy. It doesn't mean you will never experience negative emotions, or that you will feel instantly free of reactions to the seeds implanted by your past.

However, your practice can be a deep and helpful solace for you. Through the intertwining of the body, mind, psyche and reality, yoga practice can help you become compassionate, courageous and resilient. The practices can lift you out of a state of pervasive dissatisfaction and can ease a mind that is chronically ill at ease. The postures, the breathing, the relaxations and meditations can all shine sunlight for you on those days when you feel hurt, raw or struck by cosmic sadness. They can embrace you in times of quiet desperation or unconscious despair. They can cup your heart in the depths of grief, support you through trauma and hold your hand when you are on the edge. In the most natural and wholesome way, yoga can reconnect you to who you truly are.

Yoga restores our relationship to being. Whether or not we experience it as such, we all start from wholeness. So during our Hatha practices, our breathwork, our relaxations and our meditations, we proceed from wholeness. And we return to wholeness. How beautiful to realize that you are already perfect, and at the end of the day you can be present to life as it unfolds.

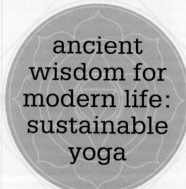

ancient wisdom for modern life: sustainable yoga

AHIMSA अहिंसा

Modern yoga is kind. The first ethical principle (*yama*) of Hatha yoga is that of *ahimsa*, which is often translated as non-violence or non-harming, so it's easy to think of it as the avoidance of aggression. However, *ahimsa* runs deeper than simply avoiding hurtful behaviour. *Ahimsa* also encompasses kindness, compassion and acceptance.

While it's uncomfortable for us to admit it, violence is a part of human nature. You can see it in a toddler's tantrum. You can see it in relationship breakdowns, or in grown-ups at war. We all have within ourselves the potential to be aggressive, unkind and violent toward ourselves and others. However, as our relationships interconnect us all, it's in your own interest to learn how to cultivate being kind to yourself, and to practise extending this kindness toward others.

While you may at times feel powerless to change the violence in the outside world, what you can do is ensure that it's not a reflection of what lies within. You can clean up your own act and consider your thoughts and actions in the light of *ahimsa*. To develop compassion and empathy, a really useful practice is the Loving-Kindness Meditation (see page 372). In this classic Buddhist practice you fill yourself with the energy of loving kindness, so that you'll have it in abundance to share with others. Then you share it out with other beings.

The precept of *ahimsa* includes not harming nature. Environmental sustainability is vital, so cut pollution,

अहिंसा

recycle and reduce consumption. Remember back in kindergarten, when you learned the difference between wants and needs? Reconsider your purchases in this light, to limit the greediness that our materialistic world encourages.

Your modern yoga practice needs to be sustainable, too. You need to ensure that your practice meets your needs and nourishes you. Modern yoga understands that correct alignment is essential to a sustainable practice. For example, check that you're not setting your shoulders up for a burnout situation, due to repeated push-ups or incorrect alignment. Modern yoga is dynamic, and your practice will change according to your needs and moods.

In a modern yoga practice you get to choose how much you work in each pose, and how much you relax within it. There will be days when the kindest thing you can do for yourself is to take it easy and include lots of restorative options and relaxation in your practice. As your body is constantly being rebuilt, the body you practise yoga with today is different from the body you practised with yesterday – there are a whole lot of new cells there, which have been created with a fresh, positive attitude.

Getting to know who we are requires non-judgement, compassion and curiosity. It also requires acceptance of body and mind. *Ahimsa* encompasses complete self-acceptance at a very deep level. In this light, you don't need to change anything at all. What is it like to realize you are already perfect?

Part 2

YOGA BODY: YANG — THE ACTIVE PRACTICES

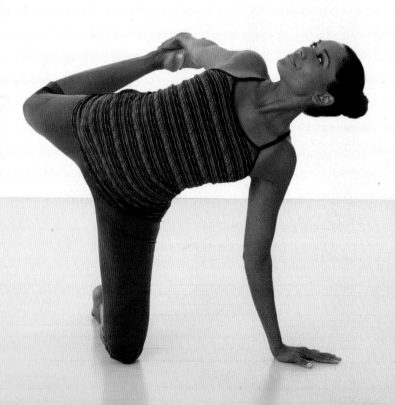

LUSCIOUS LIMBERING

I can't speak highly enough of the yogic limbering practices. As they are often less demanding physically than other poses, it means the breathing can relax and open. This is invaluable for the health of both body and mind. Limbering sequences are frequently used as preliminary practices, preparing the body for some tougher work to come, but any of these sequences are equally lovely to insert – in a kind of "less is more" way – throughout your practice. They will help to re-centre you, and you will enjoy the fact that they can be all-engrossing and yet non-demanding, in this crazy-fast world of high expectations. They can also help settle your body at the end of a workout, allowing you to slip into serenity using your relaxation or meditation techniques.

Pep yourself up with one or two of these practices during a busy workday and you'll revive your tired mind and soothe your soul. These manageable sequences are suitable for just about everybody's body, and a selection of them can create a complete practice, too (see Putting It All Together on page 376). Remember not to confuse intensity with the *quality* of your yoga practice. Just because these sequences are gentle, that doesn't mean they are not sophisticated and valuable for every single yoga practitioner. I hope you enjoy these mini-workouts as much as I do.

☆ circle of joy

What's not to love about this beautiful heart-opening sequence? Your breathing will slow and deepen, increasing the vital capacity of your lungs and building your "bank account" balance of pranic energy. And your spine will lengthen and maintain flexibility, as it arcs forward and back, keeping you feeling fresh, light and young – and, yes, joyful.

1. Sit on your heels with your big toes touching and your knees wide apart. Bring your palms together in prayer. This first time, before you begin to move, take some time to notice the shape of your spine as you sit here. Observe how your tailbone tucks lightly under, then notice the sacrum bone – that broad plate of bone leading to your lower back. Enjoy the long inward arch of your lower back, and how the mid- and upper back round softly outward. Finally, notice how your neck curves inward a little. Enjoy the way your head balances easily on the very top vertebrae. Just acknowledging these parts can allow tensions to melt away.

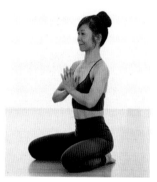

2. Take a breath in, then interlace your fingers and, turning your palms forward, exhale as you press away through the heels of the hands. At the same time, use your abdominals to help you tuck your tailbone under strongly, then round your upper back. Really go for it, with this action. Press out actively with your palms to help you cleave the shoulder blades away from each other. You want to create the maximum distance between your upper back vertebrae and your hands.

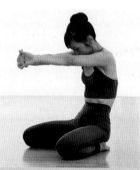

move forward
East–West Flow (page 48)

balance out
Spine Mobilizer (page 50)

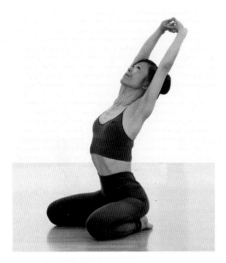

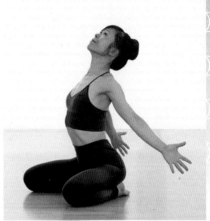

3. Catch the wave of your next inhalation and sweep your arms up to vertical, or even further back, reaching beyond vertical. As you do this, change the shape of your spine to a long concave shape. Strongly tilt your pelvis forward. Your chestbone will lift as you create a tall backbend and you will feel a great shoulder stretch. You want to enliven the whole of your spine, so focus on doing a little less with the neck vertebrae while feeling more in the spine from the neck down.

4. As you exhale, take your arms and fingers out wide to the side. Keep your spine in a backbend shape and reach the arms as far back as possible, to get a stretch across the chest muscles. Make the movement slow, so that it lasts as long as your entire exhalation does. Inhale again as you float your palms together in prayer in front of your chest. As your spine returns to its normal four curves, allow the softness to come into it and into the whole body. Repeat this breathing sequence five to ten more times.

unwind
Reclining Twist Flow (page 40)

take care
If you can't kneel comfortably, take a different seated position or stand up.

CIRCLE OF JOY

☆ tiger flow

This modern take on the classic Cat and Cow poses will mobilize your spine and bring it alive. This sequence includes triceps-toning, to keep the arms looking slender. It prepares the shoulders for the Strengthening Sun Salutation (see page 76).

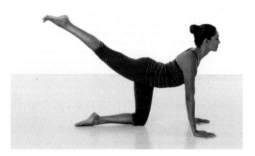

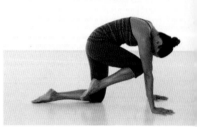

1. Begin on all fours. Inhale and take your right leg back and up, so it reaches as high up as possible. At the same time, curve your spine into a downward arch as you feed your chest through your upper arms. Allow your neck vertebrae to join the rest of the spine in this backbend, but as the neck is already flexible, place your mental emphasis more on the rest of the spine, particularly the thoracic vertebrae of the mid- and upper back.

2. Exhale as you round the spine in the opposite direction and bring your right knee into your chest. Feel your abdominals drawing inward, toward the spine, as you push the floor away with your hands. Continue for several rounds. Inhale to concave your spine. Exhale to curve it up with your right leg, reaching out like the tail of a tiger, then drawing in.

move forward
Hip-Freeing Dog to Plank (page 66)

balance out
Spine Mobilizer (page 50)

3. Add the arm-strengthening work from the backbend position, with your leg still lifted behind. To work your triceps, ensure your inner-elbow creases are facing forward, then bend both elbows backward and lower them toward the floor. Ensure both upper-arm bones are parallel as you do this, and that the elbows do not splay apart. Straighten your arms, keeping your right foot at exactly the same height as it was, so that you get a beautiful squeezy feeling in the kidney area. Keep your hip position fixed – check your hips are not moving backward as you lower yourself down (you won't feel that good triceps-muscle burn if they are). Complete eight push-ups, exhaling down and inhaling up. Then bring the knee into the chest once again before lowering it down to the floor. You are now ready for your left side.

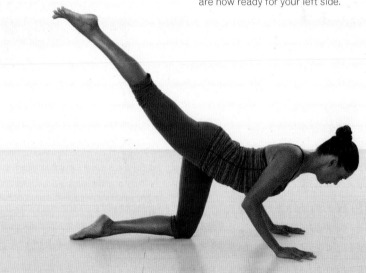

unwind
Corkscrew Twist (page 172)

take care
If your wrists need extra care, work with your fists to the floor instead of the flat of your hands.

☆ shoulder sweeps

This flow is one of my all-time favourites, not only because it's a nice shoulder-softener, but also because it enlivens the whole torso. The twisting action nicely stretches out the accessory breathing muscles around the ribs, shoulders and neck. This invites the breathing to truly open and flow. I appreciate how gentle and yet profound it is, and hope you feel it, too.

1. Start on your hands and knees. Reach your right fingertips out to the floor in front and take a slow breath in.

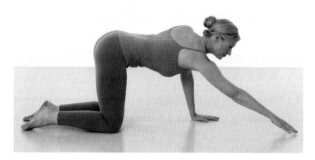

2. As you exhale, slowly slide your fingertips back past your knee. At the same time, move your hips toward your heels. Take the whole length of your exhalation to do this movement. You are not at your work desk now – remember: moving fast in yoga is not more efficient. Take your time and enjoy the lazy exhalation.

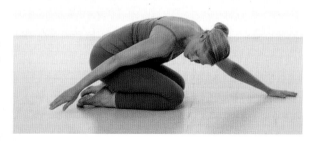

move forward
Mini Sun Salute (page 70)

balance out
Classic Downward-Facing Dog Pose
(page 58)

LUSCIOUS LIMBERING

3. When you feel your inhale begin, lift your right hand up into the air and rise up onto your knees again. Create a huge circle, to return your fingers to their starting position on the floor out in front. Exhaling, begin your next circle by sliding backward once again. Lock your gaze onto your moving thumb for the whole circle. As your right arm approaches the vertical, push your left palm firmly down and see if you can feel the rebound "bounce" that enables your right arm to reach one notch higher. Continue for five or more rounds. Then sit up and feel the difference in the two halves of your torso. Most likely your right side will feel looser, warmer, more open and relaxed.
Repeat on the left side.

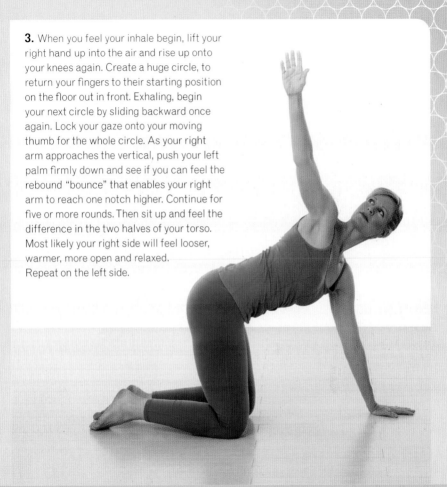

unwind
Pigeon Limbering (page 54)

wide-legged forward flow

It's a joy to feel the body loosening as you nudge it a little deeper into the release with each revisit. Besides working the backs of the legs, this sequence will also ease out any tightness in the lower back.

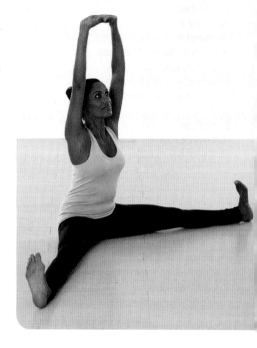

1. Sit with your legs apart in a V-shape. Before you start to move, press your hands onto the floor behind your hips and rotate your pelvis into a forward tilt. Then try removing your hands. If you find your pelvis just tilts backward, bend your knees up as much as you need to, to comfortably maintain this forward tilt for the entire sequence. You will be able to straighten them a little more toward the end. If it's easy to maintain your anterior pelvic tilt, play with anchoring yourself during the sequence by keeping the backs of your knees pressed toward the earth and flexing your feet, to pull your toes back toward your torso.

Inhale and interlace your fingers, reaching your arms forward and all the way up. Press the heels of the hands away. Enjoy the sensations of your back muscles squeezing, and notice how your heart centre elevates.

build up	move forward	balance out
Mini Sun Salute (page 70)	Deep Forward Bend at the Wall (page 152)	Cobbler's Bridge (page 192)

LUSCIOUS LIMBERING

2. Now exhale and tip your whole torso forward as you bend your elbows to float your interlaced fingers just in front of the chest. Still on that same exhalation, reach your arms forward as you fold from the hips into a forward bend.

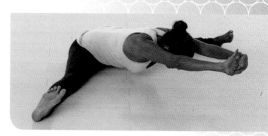

3. Inhale and contract your abdominal muscles as you bend the elbows again, to bring your hands near the heart and then reach them up overhead. Then exhale, revolve your abdomen to the right side and, still on the same long exhalation, drop the hands down to chest level and then reach both arms and torso forward over your right leg. Try to line up your chestbone with your thigh bone. Don't drop the head; instead, reach out and away through the crown of the head every time you fold forward.

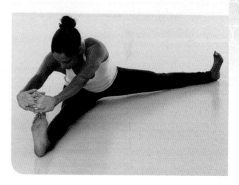

4. Inhale to come up and de-rotate, and lift to extend the crown and the palms up to the sky. Exhale as you fold forward again, torso between the thighs. Then breathe in to come up and, on your next exhale, twist left and fold over your left leg. Inhale to return to centre. Exhale to fold forward again.

Continue working through the centre and the sides, four times each. To take the load off the lower back, bend the elbows, so that the hands travel near your heart as you move into and out of each forward bend. Then take your hands to the floor to hold in each of the three forward positions for five breaths.

unwind
Resting Pigeon (page 294)

take care
If you have sacroiliac joint dysfunction, always allow your weight to shift from side to side slightly as you twist. When you twist to the right, your left buttock will slide slightly forward and lighten its weight on the floor; and the reverse when you twist left.

☆ flying locust

This pose is a must if you sit for long hours at a desk. It strengthens the back muscles and stabilizes the shoulder girdle. The first stage also neatly "tricks" the abdominals into working well, and as a result the vertebral column maintains good alignment. This will help support the spine during the second stage, which develops your flexibility in backbending.

1. From all fours, reach your right arm out so that your hand touches the floor in front, thumb up. Extend your left leg out behind you, with the toes tucked under, touching the floor.

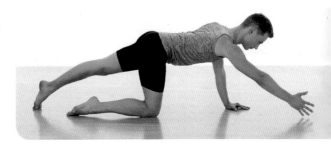

2. Inhale to prepare and then, on an exhalation, lift your right arm and left leg up to horizontal. As you lift both limbs, draw your abdominal muscles in, to lift your belly away from the floor. This will stop your lower back drooping down and will keep a sense of length in the lumbar spine.

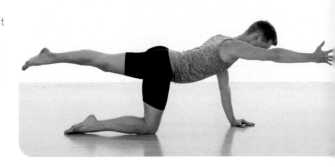

LUSCIOUS LIMBERING

move forward
Your choice of Sun Salutation (pages 68–79)

balance out
Kinky Cobbler's Pose (page 154)

3. Inhale to lower the right little finger to the floor and the left toes, then exhale to lift them again, staying mindful not to allow the belly to slacken toward the floor. Exhaling while lifting the limbs may feel a bit counter-intuitive, but it will help activate the abdomen and stabilize the pose. Repeat six rounds as you inhale to touch down, then exhale to lift up again. While the arm extends out and away, be sure to anchor the top of the arm into its root, creating a feeling of bringing the head of the upper arm bone into the shoulder girdle. Draw your right shoulder blade down toward your left hip to accentuate this feeling.

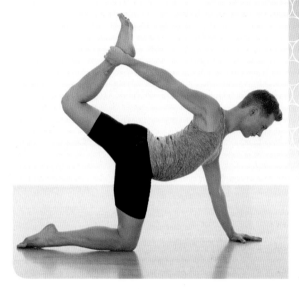

4. Progress to Kneeling Bow Pose. Bend your left knee and reach your right arm back to catch your foot. Lift your foot high in the air. Allow your spine to move into a deep back-bend. Your lower back already knows how to bend backward, so mentally emphasize the backbend in the thoracic spine. Move your chestbone forward and up. Then lift the left foot higher, to feel more of a stretch in your quadriceps. After five to ten long breaths, come out. You are now ready for side two.

unwind
Spine-Mobilizing Lunge (page 42)

take care
Use your fists on the floor if that works better for your wrists; lift only one limb at a time to make it easier.

☆ reclining twist flow

One really special thing about twists done lying down is that the spine can more easily stay l-o-o-o-o-n-g. The back muscles don't have to work hard at holding you upright and there is no downward pressure from gravity, so you get a better twist. Yum!

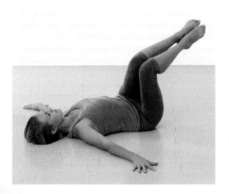 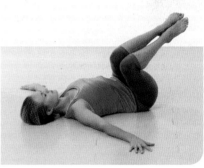

1. Lie on your back with your knees bent in, feet in the air. Switch on your abdominal muscles to bring your thighs closer to your belly. Take your arms straight out to the sides, palms down. Exhale to move both legs toward the right. Start small, so that your knees are still floating in the air. Inhale as you bring your legs back up to symmetry. Exhale and move to the left. Continue exhaling down and inhaling up, alternating sides.

move forward
Three-Step Reclining Twist (page 170)

balance out
Yin Happy Baby (page 318)

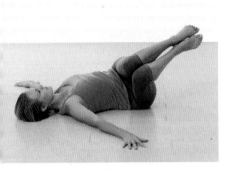

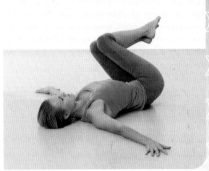

2. As your body gets warmer, you may like to travel further. It might feel good to take your legs all the way to the floor each time. Continue to work with the breath as you flow from one side to the other.

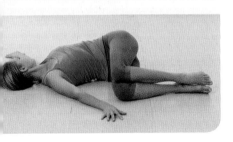

3. Come to stillness by dropping your legs all the way to the right side. If you are injury-free, it's okay if your left shoulder pops up; otherwise, try to nestle it closer to the floor. Widen the left shoulder blade away from the vertebral column and slide your left hand further away along the floor. The next part is really simple: rest and breathe. Enjoy this for a minute or more. When you are ready for side two, activate your abdominal muscles and bring your legs up, one at a time, to protect your lower back.

unwind
East–West Flow (page 48)

take care
If you have sacroiliac dysfunction, stay at step 1, avoiding the long hold.

spine-mobilizing lunge

With your knees reaching far away from each other, this pose invigorates the legs, yet invites a sort of chewing-gum softness into the pelvis and hips. It's a good example of how yin and yang – active work and enjoyable release – come together during yoga practice to give great results.

1. From all fours, step your right foot between your hands. With your front knee at a right-angle, slide your left knee back until you feel a good release in the front of the left hip. You can do this whole sequence with your back knee on the floor, and you can pad under the knee, if you like.

If you feel ready, tuck your left toes under and lift your left knee. As you do this, resist letting the hips lift. You want to *squeeze* that left knee upward, yet keep the hips low, as you reach the front knee forward more. Push down through your left palm and, as you inhale, reach your right arm out wide and up. While both knees move away from each other, so you also want to separate the distance between both hands. Look up to the top thumb and stay in this twist for several long breaths.

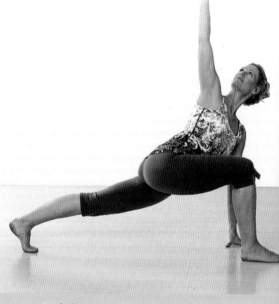

move forward
Power Squat (page 218)

balance out
Mini Sun Salute (page 70)

2. Return your right hand to the floor and lower your left knee to the floor. By now you may be ready to slide your front foot further forward. Lift your right big toe up, so that the weight rests on the outer blade of your foot. Press your right hand against the inner knee to allow it to sway out to the right side. Keep your right hand on the knee as you twist your torso deeply to the right. Lower your hips and feel the stretch in your inner right thigh. Stay for several breaths, then repeat on side two.

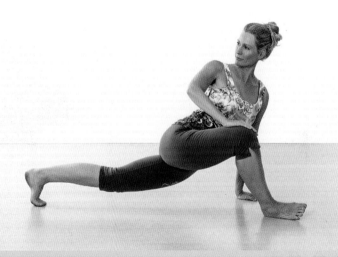

unwind
Reclining Eagle Twist (page 226)

take care
Seek further advice if you feel any discomfort in your hip joint.

gate pose with side bow

Because many yoga poses stretch the gluteal muscles, some yogis find they are lacking strength in this important stabilizing muscle group. This practice develops strength in this area, to maintain good pelvic alignment and keep your hips, knees and spine happy.

1. From a kneeling position, take your right leg straight out to the side. Position your foot so that the instep lines up with the left knee and your right toes point straight forward. Press down on the little-toe edge of the right foot, so that it is firmly anchored to the floor, almost as if you were standing normally – it's harder than it looks. Take your left palm to the floor, also in line with your left knee, fingers pointing to the left. Reach your right arm overhead, past your right ear. Stay for several long breaths, allowing the whole of the side to elongate.

move forward
Bow Pose Three Ways (page 238)

balance out
Reclining Eagle Twist (page 226)

LUSCIOUS LIMBERING

2. Now let's strengthen. Reach your right arm up to vertical. Lift your right leg up to hip height. Internally rotate your right thigh a little, so that the kneecap angles slightly downward and your toes hang toward the floor. Exhale as you lower your toes to the floor, and inhale to bring the leg up again. Repeat five to eight times.

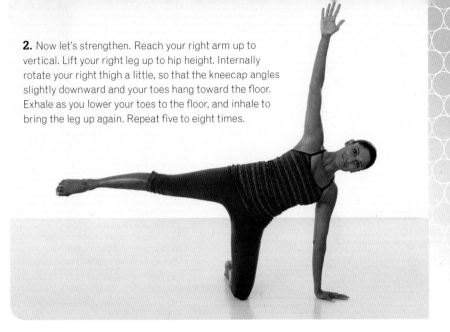

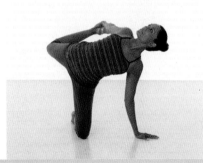

3. Develop your back-bending flexibility by bending your raised knee and reaching your top hand behind to grasp the foot. Press your right heel back away from the buttock. Enjoy the stretch in your right thigh and the front of your hip. Once you have developed your backbend shape, rotate your ribcage upward and shine that light in your heart up to the sky. Look up, if it suits your neck. Hold for five breaths. Then repeat on side two.

unwind
Pigeon Limbering (page 54)

take care
Pad underneath your kneeling knee, for greater comfort. Use a fist to the floor, if your wrist needs more support.

☆ dragon flow

This warm-up sequence is such a good package deal, as it will move your spine in all of the six directions it needs to move each day. Besides offering two twists, two side-bends, a forward bend and a backbend, it activates the core muscles; plus it strengthens the quadriceps, which will support healthy knees.

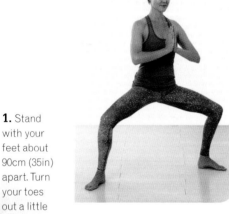

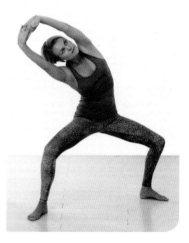

1. Stand with your feet about 90cm (35in) apart. Turn your toes out a little and slide your knees into a wide, high squat, aiming each knee over the second toe below. Start with your palms together at the chest, then inhale and interlace your fingers as you reach both arms out in front and sweep them up overhead.

2. On your next exhalation, lift your left side ribs and tilt your torso over to the right. Then inhale upright again. Exhale and side-curve toward the left. Then inhale back up again.

move forward
Dog to Plank Flow (page 210)

balance out
Shoulder-Releasing Eagle (page 116)

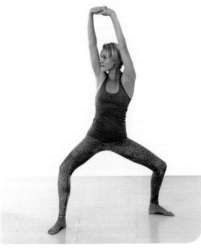

3. As you next exhale, squeeze your abdominal muscles to twist your torso to the right. In many yoga positions your arms are available to help you twist deeper, but not here. So grab this abdominal-strengthening opportunity and squeeze on your core muscles to swivel as far as you can. Inhale to return to the middle, then exhale and twist to the left before breathing in to return to the middle.

4. Now exhale to sweep your arms wide out to the side and down. Interlace your fingers behind your back. Inhale and lift the chest, to create a backbend. Get a better shoulder stretch by lifting the hands higher. Straighten your legs and move your big toes closer together, so that the outer edges of your feet are parallel. Exhale and fold forward, while you take your hands overhead, still interlaced. Stay in this wide-legged forward fold for several breaths. Inhale to return to upright, bending the knees if you need to protect your back. Swivel the feet to turn the toes out and bend your knees once again. Return the hands to a prayer pose and repeat the sequence, this time moving toward the right side first. Then do two more complete rounds.

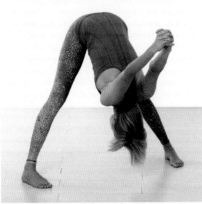

unwind
Pigeon Pose with Scientific Stretching (page 224)

take care
As you twist to the left, your right knee will tend to sag inward. Reinforce its position by pressing the back knee wider, as you take the twist.

east–west flow

This sequence stretches the back of the body (the west side, as yoga is traditionally done facing the rising sun) and the front of the body, too (the east side). While you can make the forward fold as soft and easy as you like, the lift up requires strength and builds character. Use it as an opportunity to bring constancy to the breath.

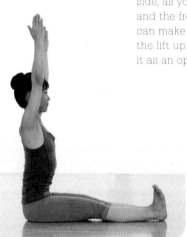

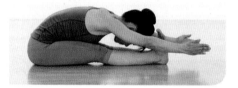

1. Sit with your legs together, extended out in front. Inhale as you reach the arms forward and up. Feel your back muscles activate, and switch on your triceps (underarm) muscles.

2. Wait for your exhalation and use it to sweep the arms and your torso forward. Don't be concerned about how far your hands reach. Think "out" rather than "down", so instead of aiming your forehead to your legs, send your energetic reach outward through the top of your head. This will create the sense of lengthening the spine from the tailbone toward the crown and will maintain a better alignment.

move forward
Mini Sun Salute (page 70)

balance out
Spine Mobilizer (page 50)

LUSCIOUS LIMBERING

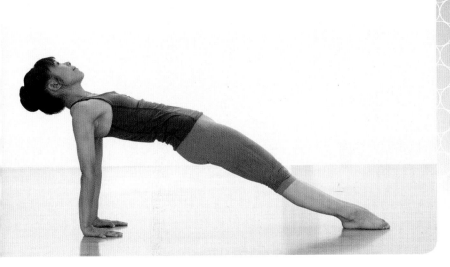

3. On your next inhalation, activate your abdominal muscles and sweep your torso and arms up. Then, as you exhale, place your palms on the floor behind your hips. Your fingers can point either forward or backward. Point your toes, inhale and lift your hips and heart forward and up. Resist the urge to drop the head all the way back. Instead, keep a sense of connection from chin to throat, so that you feel some muscle activation in your throat. With straight knees, press the big-toe knuckles down strongly and roll your thighs inward toward each other. Exhale and lower your hips to the floor. You are now ready to inhale and take your arms up once again. Repeat five to ten times.

unwind
Circle of Joy (page 30)

take care
If the hip lift feels too strong, slide your feet in a little, then bend your knees as you come up, so that your feet are flat on the floor and your body forms a table shape.

spine mobilizer

This is one of my favourite limbering sequences. The seated position subtly softens the hips and is manageable for even the tightest of hips. It feels as if the joints in the torso ease off some of their "rust", and good breathing allows the lungs to clear the "dust". And then the heart feels happier. At the end of the day, isn't that what it's all about?

1. Sit with your left shin in front of you and bend your right knee back, so that your heel is near your right hip. Snuggle your right sitting bone down to the floor. Inhale and raise both arms up overhead, and sense your spine lifting tall. Exhale and, keeping the length in the spine, float your arms down and twist to your left. Place your right hand on your left knee and take your left fingertips to the floor behind you. Use pressure on both hands to ease deeper into the twist.

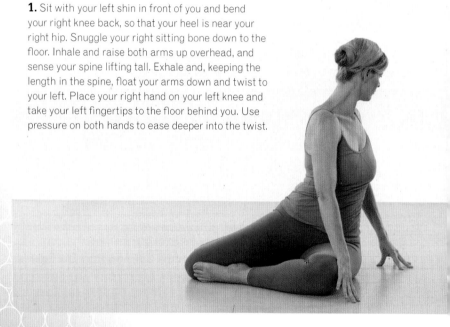

move forward
Classic Downward-Facing Dog Pose (page 58)

balance out
Hip-Releasing Wide Child Pose (page 216)

LUSCIOUS LIMBERING

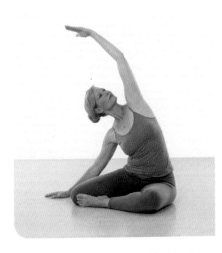

2. Get ready for the lateral stretch. Inhale your arms up overhead again. Exhale and bring your right hand to the floor, wide of your right foot, and increase the curve toward the right by reaching actively through to the top hand. Now set up your beautiful flow. Inhale as you bring your arms overhead again. Exhale as you twist left. Inhale to come out again and exhale straight into the side-bend. Continue for five more rounds.

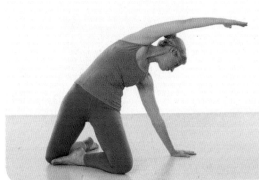

3. Finally lift into a longer hold, to stretch the front of the hips. From your last side-bend, take your left hand back around, as if to return to the twist. Press the floor away with your left hand as you extend your right arm up and back, lifting your hips in the air. Press your hips forward and lift your chest. Stay for five breaths. Then repeat on side two.

unwind
Circle of Joy (page 30)

take care
For the health of your knees, ensure that the toes of your bent back leg point backward rather than out to the side. The top of your foot will be touching the floor. The flowing part of this sequence can also be practised in a kneeling or cross-legged position.

three-step shoulder release

This is a quick way to bring fresh blood flow into chronically tight shoulders. As it is an upright posture, you can sneak this shoulder-soother into your day just about anywhere, to give those tight shoulders a break. It's a nice blend of work and release, too, as your mind asks the legs to work strongly, yet requests the shoulders to soften.

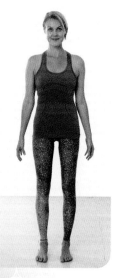

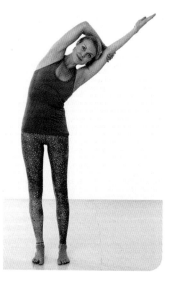

2. Reach your arms up overhead. Bend your right arm to grasp your left elbow. If possible, position your right forearm behind your head, but try to keep your neck and head in a neutral position. Anchor yourself to the earth by pressing down through the soles of your feet. Work the legs by activating your front thigh muscles to lift your kneecaps. Take a long inhalation and extend from your ankle bones all

1. Stand with your feet hip-width apart and your arms by your side in Mountain Pose.

the way up to your elbows. Feel the two side-lines of your body come alive. Continue the reach up to your left fingers. As you exhale, sway your torso to the left. Increase the shoulder stretch by moving your left arm away from your left ear.

move forward
Easy Sun Salute (page 72)

balance out
Cow-Pose Spirals (page 222)

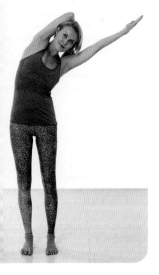

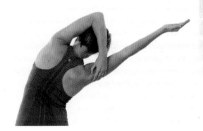

3. Inhale to come up to standing again. Exhale as you move your right hand down a little to grasp the middle of the left upper arm. Inhale to grow tall, and once again exhale to curve to the left. Sway your arm as far wide as possible. Remember to imprint your feet nicely into the ground.

Inhale to come back up. If possible, grasp your left deltoid (shoulder-cap) muscles with your right hand. If your head has been pressed forward, move the back of the skull backward to realign your head to neutral. Inhale, grow tall again, then exhale and for the third time lean to the left. Reach out with your left arm and sway it away from the head. Inhale to lift up and return to standing in Mountain Pose, with the arms by your side. Take some time to notice how and where your body has released, before you start side two.

unwind
Tension-Releasing Forward Fold (page 156)

take care
Seek advice from your physical therapist if you have pain raising your arms overhead.

☆ pigeon limbering

This is such a relaxing way to limber up tight hips. I also enjoy how the back subtly stretches as the spine rounds – it's as if the lower back breathes a sigh of relief. As the back and hips release, the breath is encouraged to lengthen, inviting your mind to release its tensions, too.

LUSCIOUS LIMBERING

1. Begin on all fours. With an inhalation, hover your right knee in the air to bring it forward between your hands. Have it far enough forward that your right foot is able to clear your left knee.

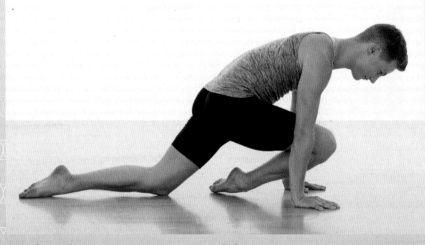

move forward
Twisted Pigeon (page 182)

balance out
Cobbler's Bridge (page 192)

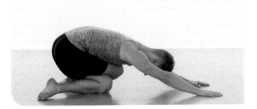
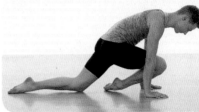

2. Exhale and slide your right foot down the left side of your left shin to stack your right knee in front of your left knee. As you perform this sliding action, take your buttock back to your left heel. Curve your tailbone under and lift your lower and middle back toward the sky. With your hips settled back and down, you will feel a stretch in the left buttock area.

3. Inhale to return your right knee between your hands, ready for the next movement. Take the rounding out of your spine, so that it's in a more neutral position, with a light abdominal contraction so that your belly lifts up away from the floor.

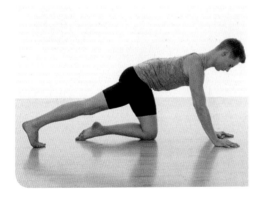

4. Exhale and lengthen your right leg away, landing your foot on the floor, toes tucked under. Press your right heel away to create a light calf stretch. Inhale to begin the next round, again moving the right leg. The movements will become noticeably more fluid and enjoyable as your body softens. Repeat for five to ten rounds. Sit back, create fists and circle your wrists a few times in both directions. Then enjoy working the left side.

unwind
Banana Pose (page 194)

take care
If the angle doesn't suit either knee in step 2, perform this action without crossing your foot to the opposite side, so that your shins stay parallel with their thighs above.

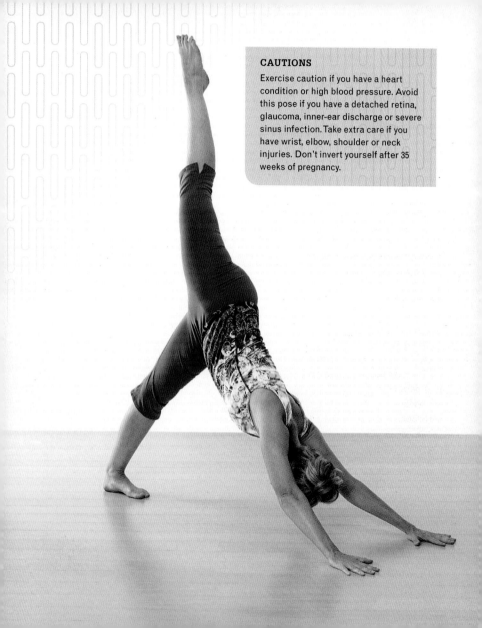

CAUTIONS

Exercise caution if you have a heart condition or high blood pressure. Avoid this pose if you have a detached retina, glaucoma, inner-ear discharge or severe sinus infection. Take extra care if you have wrist, elbow, shoulder or neck injuries. Don't invert yourself after 35 weeks of pregnancy.

DELICIOUS DOGS

The Dog is my desert-island pose – if I had to choose one from the thousands of yoga postures, I would select the simple and affectionately named Dog. A soft inversion, this pose is also an arm-strengthener, a shoulder-stretcher, a back-lengthener, a hamstring- and calf-loosener and a brain-refresher. Surely it would be greedy to ask for more from a single pose.

The Classic Downward-Facing Dog (see page 58) is a great linking pose. From any wide-legged standing pose, it's easy to cartwheel the hands to drop into Dog; do this between working on your left and right sides. And as part of a Sun Salutation, it

feels so inviting to stay and linger while you watch and steady your breath.

You can spend years developing and finessing your Dog Pose prowess. Stretching and strengthening in equal parts, this pose may highlight areas where your body is more limited. But don't be dispirited if it feels like hard work at the beginning. Keep on practising and you will find that the posture becomes less arduous and you can relax deeply in the pose. Then the rewards will be apparent, and you'll understand why this head-down triangular shape has become synonymous with yoga around the world.

classic downward-facing dog pose

Use this pose as a standalone posture, with a nice long hold or two. Or use it more briefly, as a linking posture and to help add flow and vibrancy to your practice, joining sets of standing postures.

1. You can start this pose on hands and knees, but the first few times you practise it, here's how to find out what spacing suits you best. Lie face-down on the floor. Bend your elbows up to place your palms on the floor at chest level with your thumbs at nipple level.

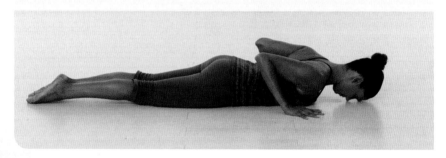

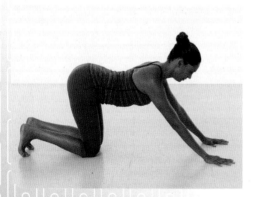

2. Without changing the position of your palms or knees, push up onto your hands and knees. With your knees and feet hip-width apart, spread your fingers and thumbs wide and tuck your toes under. Now set up the forward tilt for your pelvis for this pose, by lifting your sitting bones and letting your abdomen drop, as you accentuate the downward curve in your lower back.

3. Check that your palms are shoulder-width apart and press into the floor. Maintaining the forward pelvic tilt, lift your knees and send the hips up and back. Stay on tiptoes and keep a bend in your knees so you will be able to bring your spine to a fairly straight position. You want to send the hips energetically up away from the wrists, as far back and high as possible. Have your ears positioned between the upper arms, to keep your neck in a neutral position. Ensure that your chin is not tucked in, which would flatten the neck, and don't create any wrinkles in the back of your neck, due to over-arching it.

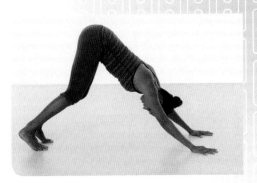

4. To maintain that lumbar curve, take your time straightening your legs and lowering the heels toward the floor. Contract your quadriceps muscles, so that the kneecaps lift. It's not the aim of this pose to have your heels on the floor: instead, aim to get maximum

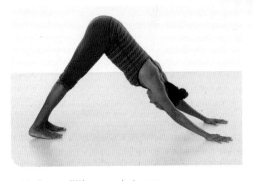

length through the back of the body. It's great to have a little space between the heels and the floor. Ensure that the index finger and thumb knuckles are well anchored down. Now roll your shoulders out, so that you broaden the shoulder blades away from each other: imagine that you have an eye in each armpit and you want to look cross-eyed. Hold and enjoy for five to ten breaths, then rest. If your wrists start to ache, then that's enough of this pose for the day; aim to build up your strength over time.

cautions
Avoid upside-down poses if you have high blood pressure, a detached retina or a risk of glaucoma.

☆ restful dogs

There's a Dog Pose for every mood. While you build strength and flexibility for longer holds in the classic Dog, here is a restful and easier option to help you enjoy your practice.

quarter-dog

This relaxing option is a great alternative to the classic Dog, if you are lower in energy or just want to give your shoulders a really good stretch-out.

1. From all fours, walk your hands forward and lower your chest as close as possible to the floor. Keep your hips above your knees and enjoy the hammocky shape of your spine. As your hips reach up and back, allow your navel and heart centres to drop down, so that you can experience the special shoulder-release.

Most people like to touch their foreheads to the floor in this pose. If you are more flexible, then you may prefer to rest one cheek to the floor. If you are even more open through the back and shoulders, you may like to rest your chin to the floor, so that you gaze forward (as long as this feels good for your neck). Rest here for five to ten breaths.

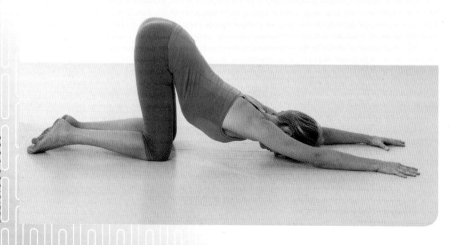

half-and-half dog

This option is for those whose arms are still building up the weight-bearing ability demanded by the classic Dog.

1. Stand with your feet wide apart and your toes pointing straight ahead. Fold over and walk your hands away, keeping them shoulder-width apart. Keep your hips directly above your ankle joints. Your upper body will be on an incline. As in a regular Dog Pose, you want to keep a long, flat feeling in your spine. In order to maintain that slight inward curve with the lumbar spine, you may do well to bend the knees; or you could place your hands on yoga bricks for a bit of height. Aim to close the gap between your armpits and the floor a little, even while you send a charge of energy through your elbows to lift them away from the floor; coming up onto your fingertips will help. Notice how long you feel through your front body, from your pubic bone to your throat. This will help you to enjoy some slow, deep inhalations and long, languid exhalations.

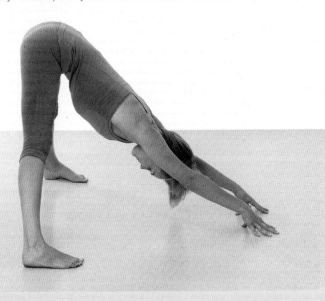

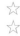

three-legged dogs

These Dog Pose variations are handy starting positions for when you want to step one foot forward between the hands, to move into a lunge-based posture or any of the standing poses.

three-legged dog

So much of yoga focuses on lengthening the hamstring muscles, but it's important that they are strong, too. This pose will strengthen one set of hamstrings as the other side lengthens.

1. From the Classic Downward-Facing Dog Pose (see page 58), lift your right leg to horizontal. Keep your hips level, so that you create a flat line from left to right across the buttocks. While your palms actively press the floor away, enjoy a lifting energy in the arms as you squeeze the arm muscles. Ensure your raised leg is truly straight by firming the muscles around the kneecap. Look back at your raised leg: check that your toes point straight down to the floor, rather than turning out to the right. This way, your right hamstrings are getting strong. Send a message to your left hamstrings to release, and lower your left heel closer to the floor.

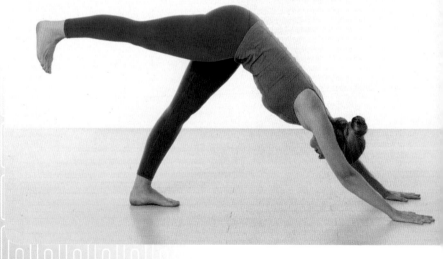

dog-pose split

What a gorgeous feeling this release in the front of the hip
gives, as you soar one leg skyward.

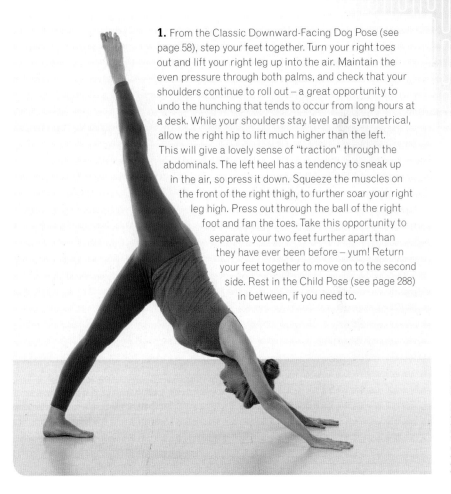

1. From the Classic Downward-Facing Dog Pose (see
page 58), step your feet together. Turn your right toes
out and lift your right leg up into the air. Maintain the
even pressure through both palms, and check that your
shoulders continue to roll out – a great opportunity to
undo the hunching that tends to occur from long hours at
a desk. While your shoulders stay level and symmetrical,
allow the right hip to lift much higher than the left.
This will give a lovely sense of "traction" through the
abdominals. The left heel has a tendency to sneak up
in the air, so press it down. Squeeze the muscles on
the front of the right thigh, to further soar your right
leg high. Press out through the ball of the right
foot and fan the toes. Take this opportunity to
separate your two feet further apart than
they have ever been before – yum! Return
your feet together to move on to the second
side. Rest in the Child Pose (see page 288)
in between, if you need to.

dogs with a twist

Add a twist to your Dog, for extra strength and stretch,
with these two fun options to liven up your practice.

spiralling dog

This strongly levered twist is very strengthening for your supporting wrist,
arm and shoulder – and your torso comes alive, too.

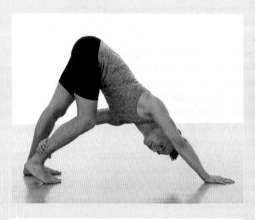

1. Take the Classic Downward-Facing Dog Pose (see p.58), but with the hands a little closer to your feet than usual. Bend your right knee and lift your right heel high in the air. Squeeze on the muscles of your right arm and press your right palm into the floor. Ensure there is plenty of pressure through the right thumb and index finger, too. Reach your left hand back toward the inside of your right leg. Hook your palm around the back of the left leg, as low down as possible. You might by grasping the upper or mid-calf at first, but in time aim for the inner heel.

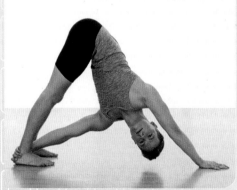

2. Now straighten your right knee and lower your right heel as much as possible. Create a spiral of energy through the torso, by reinforcing the upward reach of the right hip. Revolve your torso to the right side and look up under your armpit. Enjoy several long breaths, then practise the second side. Rest in the Child Pose (see page 288).

double-twist dog pose

The special ankle action of this pose feels as if it creates space in the hip joint, while you get a really toning twist to the torso.

1. From the Dog-Pose Split (see page 63), bend your right knee and bring the heel toward the right buttock. Strongly squeeze your thigh muscles to press your right knee up and far away. Move the ankle joint between flexion (with toes fanned) and extension (with toes pointed). After hinging at the ankle a few times, press the heel away, to hold the flexing action. Now rotate your chest and belly to the right, allowing your right shoulder to lift slightly. Tuck your chin in and look up under the right armpit. Now try twisting the less-obvious way, by turning your head and chest to the left, while dropping your right shoulder and lifting your left. If you reinforce your right hip to maintain its lift and keep reaching through the right knee, you can create a marvellous sense of release in the abdominal muscles. It can feel as if this pose is working even deeper than just on this muscular level – as if even the organs of the abdomen get more space, as they float in upside-down suspension.

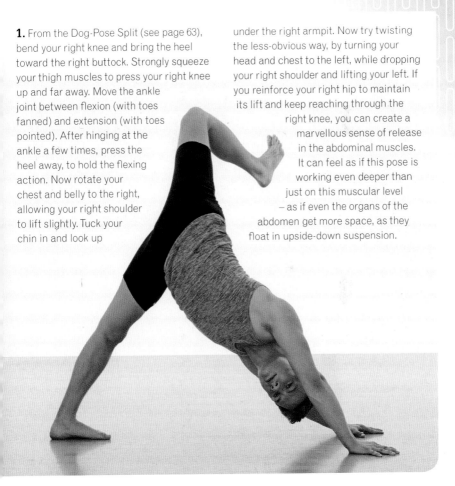

☆ hip-freeing dog to plank
☆

This flowing movement strengthens the shoulders, core and buttock muscles. If you love the figure-of-eight action of the leg, but are still developing your upper-body strength, you can work this action in an all-fours position

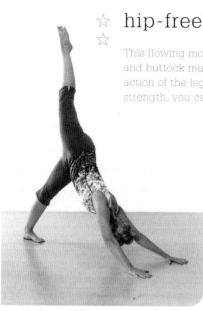

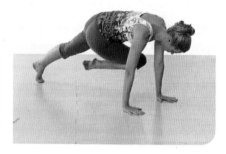

1. Start with your right leg up in the air in Dog-Pose Split (see page 63), but have your left foot several inches further away from your hands than in a usual Dog Pose. This will increase your strength when you come into the Plank position in step 2. As you inhale, reach your right leg out wide to the right side. You will need to activate the stabilizing muscles of your left buttock strongly, to prevent swaying too much to the left side.

2. As you begin your exhalation, tuck your tailbone under and bring your pelvis forward and down, to come into a Plank position. Your shoulders will now sit above your wrists. At the same time, bend your right knee and draw it across the torso toward your left armpit. Lift your abdominal muscles up toward the spine to help with this action.

build up
Seated Yogic Roll-Downs
(page 204)

move forward
Yoga Swimming Bow (page 240)

balance out
Pigeon Crescent Pose
(page 242)

DELICIOUS DOGS

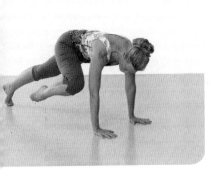

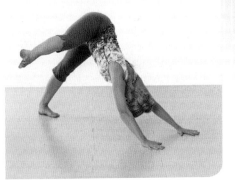

3. Still on the same long exhalation, continue the flowing leg movement by moving your right knee toward your right armpit. Create a fairly straight line from your left heel to the back of your head. Ensure there is no hinge at the hips, so that you don't droop through the front or lift through the buttocks.

4. As you inhale, complete the figure-of-eight movement, reaching your hips up and back to form an inverted V-position, as you straighten your right leg back up and away to your starting position, ready for round two. Complete four or more rounds. Then rest the knees down, sit up and ease out your wrists by circling them a few times in each direction. Then practise the second side.

unwind
Backbend Ripple (page 290)

take care
Should your wrists start to ache, ease back and build up your strength over the weeks and months. Practising a narrow Dog, with feet closer to the hands, is easier on weaker core muscles. Avoid upside-down poses if you have high blood pressure, a detached retina or a risk of glaucoma.

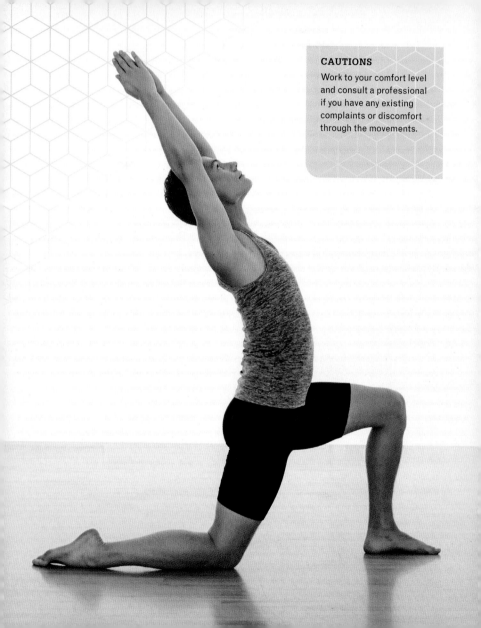

3

SUN SALUTES

There are nearly as many Sun Salute variations in the world as there are yoga teachers, and it's fun getting creative with these flowing movements. While you may prefer to stick faithfully to the routines, you can change it up too, using your Sun Salutes as a springboard to launch into your favourite standing poses.

Go with your mood as you practise. You can choose to work slowly, feeling your way into each position over the course of several breaths. Alternatively, you can develop your rhythmic flow, by performing one movement on each inhalation and exhalation, to create a moving meditation.

Each of the following Salutes has a different flavour. I hope you will find one that suits they way you're feeling – not only today, but on any given day.

☆ mini sun salute

This a great and manageable way to ensure the correct setting of your shoulders before you progress on to the Strengthening Sun Salutation (see page 76). It warms up and strengthens the arms, shoulders and core while providing a gentle back-stretch.

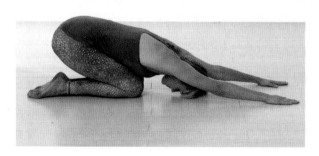

1. Kneel and lower your hips to come into the Child Pose (see page 288). Reach your arms forward, palms down, and rest your forehead on or just above the floor.

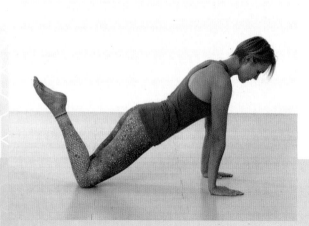

2. Rise up to a kneeling Plank position, with your shoulders over your wrists. This first time, move your knees back, to create a straight line from shoulders to knees. Lift your feet so that your toes point forward.

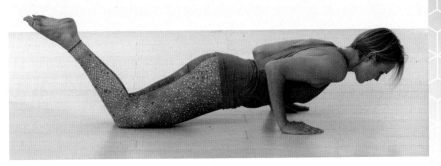

3. Create a small roll-back with your shoulders, to broaden across your collar bones. Then exhale and bend your elbows backward while you lower your torso down. There are three important moves here. The first is to magnetize your shoulder blades toward each other. If you start to roll your shoulders in, don't drop any lower, even if you have only lowered a tiny bit. Keep practising while your strength builds. Second, don't splay your elbows out to the sides. Finally, draw your abdomen toward your spine. You won't be lowering all the way to the floor, but imagine that if you were, your chest would touch down before your belly.

4. Inhale to push back up to the kneeling Plank position. Keep your abdominal muscles strongly engaged – don't sag your hips or leave your belly behind. Check that your shoulders don't roll in. If they do, don't lower so much next time.

5. Exhale and, with palms glued to the floor, curve your spine upward and take your hips back toward your heels. You may not reach all the way back to the Child Pose, but that doesn't matter. You are going for a lovely release along the sides of the torso. If you let your hands slide back toward your knees, you will lose that stretch. Wait for your next in-breath to begin the next round, and repeat for five to eight rounds.

take care
Ask a physiotherapist about weight-bearing, if you have shoulder injuries.

MINI SUN SALUTE

☆ easy sun salute

Because yoga is traditionally practised facing the east, this invigorating sequence is a great way to greet the rising sun each morning. You might begin by taking a couple of breaths in each position, then match each movement to a single inhalation or exhalation. Get into the flow of your day by completing six to eight rounds.

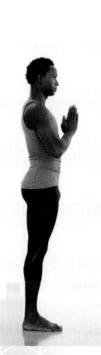 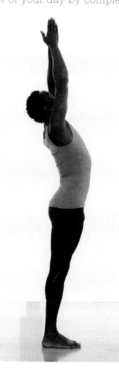 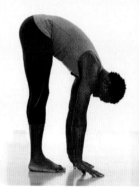

1. Stand straight with your feet hip-width apart. Take your palms together in the prayer position.

2. As you take a breath in, reach your arms forward and up overhead, and enjoy the lift and curve of your upper back.

3. On your next exhalation, fold forward from the hips and bring your hands to the floor. Bend the knees, if you need to.

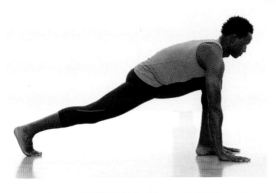

4. On an inhalation, step your right leg back into a lunge.

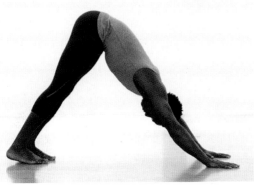

5. As you exhale, step your left leg back to create an inverted V-shaped Classic Downward-Facing Dog Pose (see page 58).

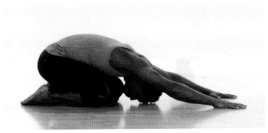

6. On an inhalation, lower both knees to the floor, and then exhale to take your hips back toward your heels and come into the Child Pose (see page 288).

Continues overleaf →

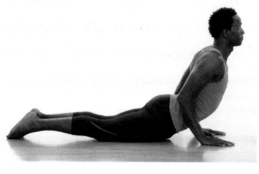

7. Look forward and then sweep your chest as low as possible between your thumbs, before curving your spine into a Cobra shape (see page 230).

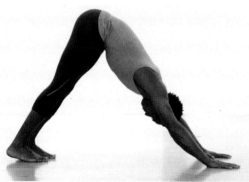

8. Take your gaze forward and draw your navel toward your spine to engage your core muscles. Then exhale and lift your hips back up to a Downward Facing Dog. If you have a tender lower back, bend the knees as you make this transition.

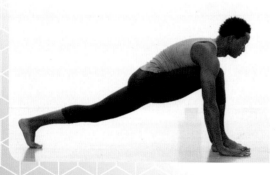

9. Look forward and lift your right wrist. While inhaling, step your right leg forward between your hands. Take an extra little hop or two forward, if you don't get all the way the first time.

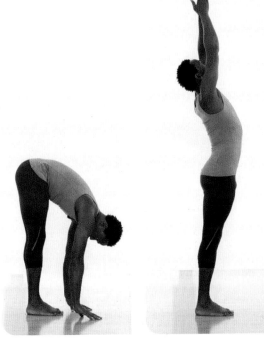
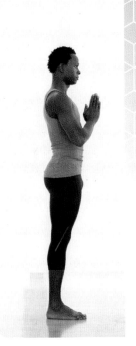

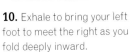
10. Exhale to bring your left foot to meet the right as you fold deeply inward.

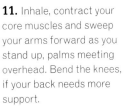
11. Inhale, contract your core muscles and sweep your arms forward as you stand up, palms meeting overhead. Bend the knees, if your back needs more support.

12. Exhale and lower your prayer-like palms to your chest. Inhale, ready to sweep the arms out to begin the next round, alternating sides so that this time your left leg steps back, then forward. Complete three to four rounds on each side.

strengthening sun salutation

☆
☆
☆

This Sun Salutation is found in Ashtanga yoga. It will warm and strengthen your whole body. Once you find your rhythm in this beautifully symmetrical sequence, you will be able to set up a nice flowing breath. It's a great basis from which to lead off into a whole sequence of standing poses.

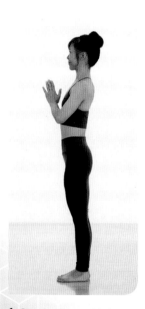 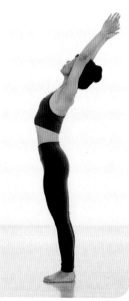 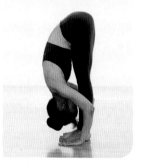

1. Stand with your big toes touching and your palms together at the centre of your chest.

2. Drop your hands by your sides, then inhale and, with palms turned upward, reach out through the fingertips to float your arms out and up. Gaze up and lift your chestbone.

3. Exhale and fold forward from the hips. As you do so, turn your palms out and sweep your arms wide, to bring your fingertips to the floor in front of your toes. Bend your knees, if you can't quite reach.

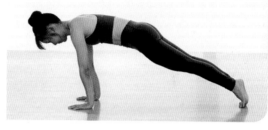

5. Exhale and, with palms flat to the floor, jump, step or walk both feet back, to create a Plank shape.

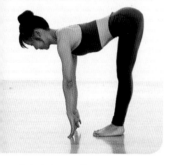

4. Inhale and flatten your spine as you gaze slightly forward. (If you can't create that hammock shape in your back, bend your knees and run your fingers up to your knees until you feel your back-muscles engage. With bent knees, return your hands to the floor, ready for the next step.)

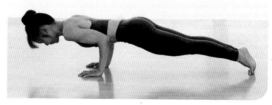

6. Still on the same exhalation, bend your elbows so they touch your sides, and lower your torso down to hover just above the floor.

Continues overleaf ➡

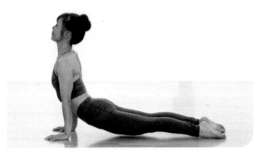

7. Engage your abdominal muscles as you inhale, and roll over your toes to shift your torso forward and up into a backbend for an Upward-Facing Dog. Roll your shoulders back and down. Keep your core and the muscles on the fronts of your thighs engaged.

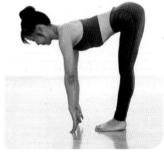

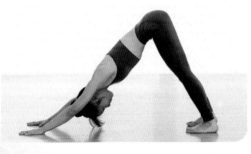

8. Exhale as you roll backward over your toes (or tuck them under, one foot at a time) and lift your hips to come into a Classic Downward-Facing Dog Pose (see page 58). Take five slow, deep breaths here.

9. After an exhale, look forward to where you want your feet to land and, with empty lungs, jump (or step) your feet between your hands. Inhale and lift your shoulders to arch the spine into a backbend shape. Broaden across your collar bones. As in step 4, bend the knees and adjust the hand position, if you need to.

move forward

Each time you find yourself in Classic Downward-Facing Dog Pose (see page 58), lunge one leg forward to complete the standing pose of your choice. Once complete, step your front leg to the back, to resume your Sun Salute flow.

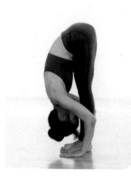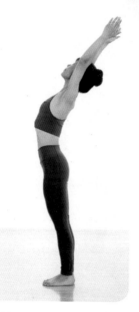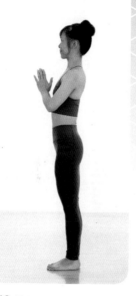

10. Exhale to fold the two halves of your body as close together as feels good.

11. Engage your abdominals, and inhale as you move your hips forward a little and lift to standing, with your palms reaching tall.

12. Exhale to return to the start, ready to repeat five or more rounds.

take care

To protect a weak back, ensure that your abdominals are engaged as you transition in and out of both Downward-Facing Dog and Upward-Facing Dog. Bend your knees as you move in and out of Downward-Facing Dog. If your shoulders need extra care, lower the knees to the floor in the Plank position, lower your legs and hips to the floor during Upward Dog, and don't hold for too long in Downward Dog.

☆ salute to the moon

This peaceful sequence is beautifully well-rounded, thanks to the twisting and side-bending actions as you make shapes that reflect the cycle of the moon. Take several breaths in each shape, or flow a little faster with one breath per movement.

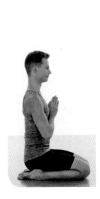 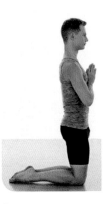 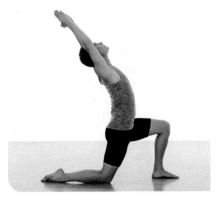

1. Kneel with your palms together at the heart.

2. Inhale as you lift your hips to a high kneel.

3. Exhale as you step your left leg forward to an easy lunge. Cross your thumbs and inhale as you sweep your arms out and up high.

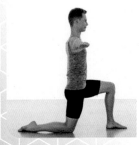 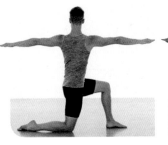

4. Exhale to bring your arms wide, to horizontal. Hold the position and breathe in as you float your spine tall.

5. Exhale and twist to the left. Inhale, returning to centre. Exhale and twist to the right. Then inhale to the middle again.

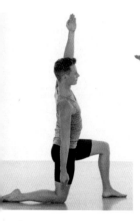

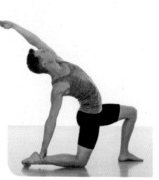

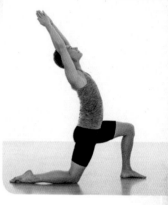

6. Exhale and drop your left arm down as you side-bend. Inhale to the centre. Exhale to reach your left arm up as you curve to the right side, then inhale up again.

7. Tuck your back toes under. Inhale and sweep both hands forward and up. Continue to circle your right hand backward until it reaches the right heel. Exhale and use the reach of your left arm to lift the heart and support the backbend.

8. Inhale to reach both arms up in the air. Then move your front leg back to a high kneeling position.

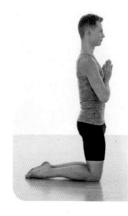

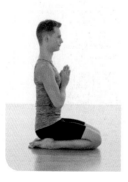

9. Exhale to return the prayer to the heart and sit down on your heels.

10. You have done half of one round. Now practise on the second side, then work with alternate sides for a total of four to six rounds.

putting it all together

☆ **15-minute quick-and-easy, all-over supple and strength set**
This short practice will refresh both body and mind. Use it as a standalone sequence or to limber up, before launching into some of the postures and practices on the following pages.

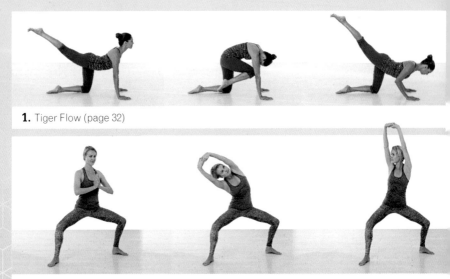

1. Tiger Flow (page 32)

3. Dragon Flow (page 46)

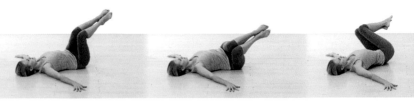

5. Reclining Twist Flow (page 40)

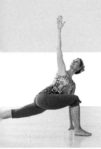
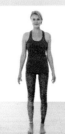

Spine-Mobilizing Lunge (page 42)

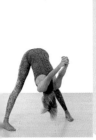
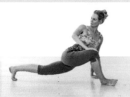
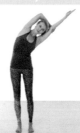
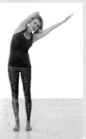

4. Three-Step Shoulder Release (page 52)

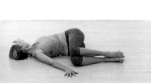
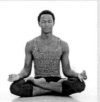

6. Mindfulness Meditation (page 366): 5 minutes

PUTTING IT ALL TOGETHER

83

complete 20-minute mini yoga practice for all ages and abilities

This stretch-and-lengthen sequence suits just about everyone. Use it morning, night or whenever you need a break during the day.

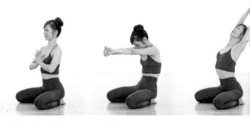

1. Circle of Joy (page 30): 5 cycles

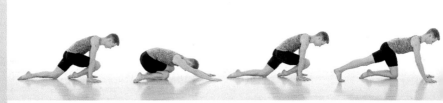

3. Pigeon Limbering (page 54): 5 on each side

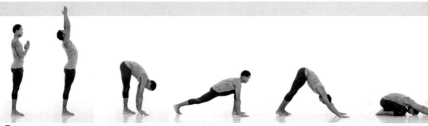

5. Easy Sun Salute (page 72–75): 3 on each side

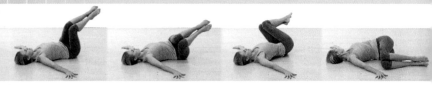

6. Reclining Twist Flow (page 40)

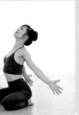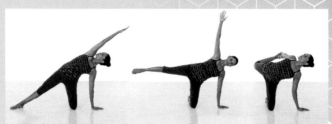

2. Gate Pose with Side Bow (page 44)

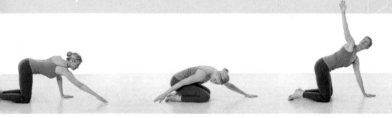

4. Shoulder Sweeps (page 34): 5 on each side

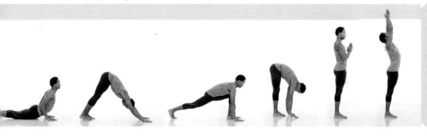

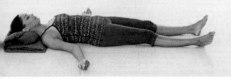

7. Peaceful Mind Relaxation (page 352): 5 minutes

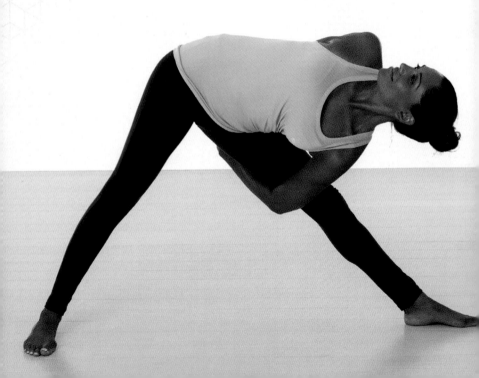

4

STABLE AND STEADY: STANDING POSTURES

Standing poses are brilliant, because even a single standing pose tends to offer you so many different openings. These are perfect positions for time-poor modern yogis, as they tick so many of the boxes that explain why people come to yoga. They give you strength. They give you flexibility. Within the standing-posture group you will meet all kinds of movements to keep you feeling loose, limber and free.

These poses offer twists, side-stretches, backbends, forward bends, balance work, core activation, hip stretches and shoulder releases. They will help you to "stand your ground" as you develop strength and stamina in your legs. They will teach you about reaching for the stars as you learn to radiate your limbs out and up. So what are you waiting for? Enjoy your journey with these multifaceted postures.

☆ chair-pose flow

This pose is great for your posture if you sit for long hours at a desk. It strengthens the back muscles and works the legs. Adding in the Ocean Breath (see page 332) will bring a constancy to the rate of your flowing movements. It will also declutter your mind, by moving your focus into the present moment. That's when true yoga practice begins and magic happens.

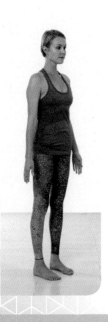

1. Stand with your feet hip-width apart. Check your feet position and make sure that both second toes are pointing forward. With your arms by your side, allow the shoulders to just fall away from the ears. This is the Mountain Pose.

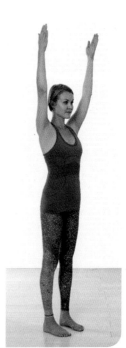

2. Inhale as you take your arms out to the sides and reach them up. Finish with your palms overhead, shoulder-width apart and facing forward.

build up	move forward	balance out
Shoulder Sweeps (page 34)	Revolved Bound Lunge (page 92)	Shoulder-Releasing Forward Fold (page 108)

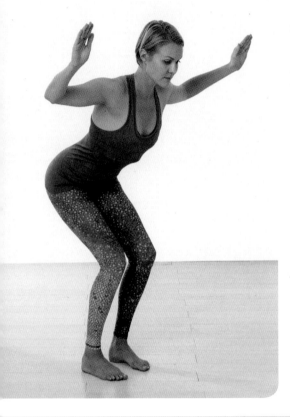

3. Now exhale as you bend your knees to take your hips back and down, as if you were about to sit on a chair, but decided to hover over it instead. While your knees will move forward as they bend, minimize this by ensuring that you are taking plenty of weight through your heels. You may even feel your toes wanting to lift up, but keep them anchored. These movements will strengthen the fronts of your thighs. At the same time, bend your elbows wide as you lower them. Ease your upper-arm bones backward until you feel your upper-back muscles working. Inhale to return to step 2, with your straight arms reaching overhead. Exhale and lower your arms to return to the Mountain Pose. Inhale to begin the next round and repeat for five to eight rounds in total.

unwind
Heavenly Happy-Baby Pose (page 158)

take care
Keep your neck in its natural curve. Resist any tendencies to jut the chin forward or to over-flatten the neck, with a big tuck-in of the chin.

☆ warrior I breathing flow

The flowing movement of this exercise will keep your breathing smooth, so the strong working of the leg, back and shoulder muscles won't feel as intense. This will keep you going longer so that you can get stronger and stronger.

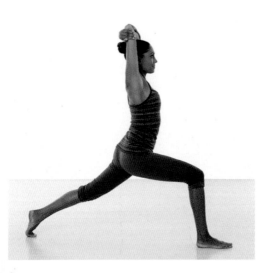

1. From standing, step your right foot forward about 1.2–1.5m (4–5ft). With your left heel lifted, bend your right knee to 90 degrees, so that you are in a high lunge. Reach your arms up overhead and cup the elbows in the palm of your hands. Next, create a tucking-under action with your tailbone to increase the stretch in the front of your left hip. Reinforce your back knee lift, so that it doesn't sag, while you maintain this pelvic tucking-under action. Now finesse this a bit: starting from just above the hips, lift up through the sides of your torso so that your forearms move away from the crown of the head. As you do this, anchor the shoulder blades downward so that the shoulders don't hunch, but everything else will have a sense of squeezing upward. While your upper body continues to lift, create your anchoring with the lower half of your body: from your hips, extend back and out strongly through the left heel. By increasing the distance between the back heel and both elbows, you will create a delicious feeling of length.

build up	**move forward**	**balance out**
Flying Locust (page 38)	Half-Frog, Half-Locust (page 236)	Shoulder-Releasing Forward Fold (page 108)

2. On an exhalation, plug in your abdominals by drawing your navel toward your spine, and lean your torso forward. Let the strong sheets of muscles over your back activate, keeping your back feeling flat and strong. Do not drop your arms – hold your upper arms level with your ears. Inhale and return to the first position, then set up your flow by moving with each part of your breath: inhaling upright, and exhaling to lower. Repeat for five to ten rounds.

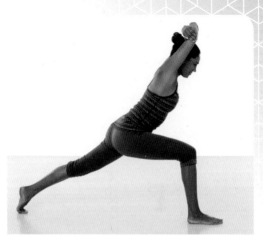

3. Now build your stamina and strength by strategically increasing the load on your upper-back muscles. Hold your forward tilt and straighten your arms, with palms facing each other, shoulder-width apart. Hold still in this position for five to ten breaths. Reinforce the posterior pelvic-tucking-under action and work through the points in step 2 to enhance the posture. Then change legs and complete the second side.

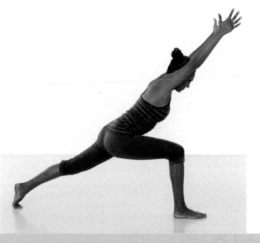

unwind
Restorative Twist (page 292)

take care
If you feel any discomfort in the lower back, don't lift so upright, but keep some forward lean in steps 1 and 2. Be conscientious about keeping the core muscles on, too.

revolved bound lunge

The arms are powerful drivers, which really help to enliven the spine in this twisting sequence. As this requires a bit more balance than you may think, it will develop poise, too.

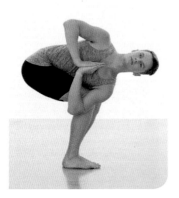

1. Stand with your feet together and your palms touching, in prayer. On an exhale, come into a squat. Inhale and lift your chestbone to touch your thumbs. Now exhale and twist to the right, and lodge your left elbow close to your outer right knee. If you can't lock your elbow in place, bring your torso up a little higher, take your left hand to your outer right knee and place your right hand on your right hip instead. Tuck your chin in slightly and look up. If your palms are together, bring the elbows to a 90-degree bend, if possible, so that your hands move closer to your hip. You can then "drive" your right palm downward while you resist with the left. This will rotate your torso further into the twist. Stay for several long breaths, then progress to the lunge.

2. Looking down, lift your left heel. If you can, lift the whole foot to hover in the air. Send your leg back to take a long, deep lunge position. Continue pressing the palms together to allow the torso to twist deeply.

build up	**move forward**	**balance out**
Threaded Needle (page 180)	Revolved Happy Pose (page 174)	Yin Happy Baby (page 318)

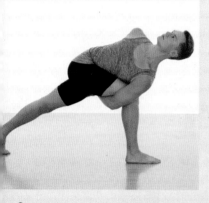
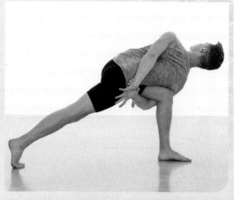

3. If you can, bring the shoulders into play. Lean further forward and lower your left shoulder to lock against your right outer knee. Bending at the elbow, rotate your left palm backward, then slide the back of the hand under your right thigh. Reach your right arm up to vertical, and turn from the shoulder so that the thumb points downward. Bring that arm down past the lower back and catch the fingers or grasp the right wrist. Looking up, deepen the twist by attempting to straighten your elbows. Reach your knuckles away so that your hands no longer touch your body. Stay for five breaths, then repeat on the second side.

unwind
Reclining Eagle Twist
(page 226)

take care
If are overly lax in either sacroiliac joint, don't try to keep your knees together in step 1. Rather, allow your left knee to slide forward of the right one, so that instead of restraining your left hip, it will move forward into the twist with you.

expansive breath warrior

I just love how strong and sharp the lines of energy feel in both steps of this Warrior practice, and how you can really imagine the capacity of your lungs expanding, as they respond to your upward reaches. Try it out and feel for yourself.

1. Step your feet about 1.2m (4ft apart). Turn your left foot out so that the toes point away from your body and move your right foot so that it points inward by about 15 degrees. Now take your arms up to join the palms overhead. Create a nice feeling in the shoulders by broadening across your upper back and moving the outer edges of your armpits slightly toward each other. Press down actively into the floor with your feet. Lift your kneecaps by pulling them up with your front thigh muscles, so that the legs feel super-strong and steady. Enhance the lift upward by elevating your ribcage away from your hips. Next, reach your elbows higher up in the air, then lengthen all the way through to your fingertips. Exhale as you turn your palms outward and widen your arms

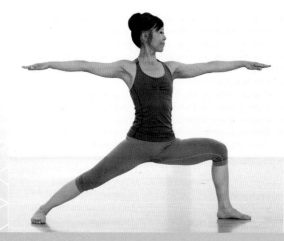

to horizontal. At the same time, bend your left knee, bringing your thigh bone to horizontal, or as close to that as is manageable. Adjust your foot spacing as needed on this first round. Anchor through your back foot and keep your back leg feeling active. Check your front knee tracks over your second toe and that your knee is above – and not in front of – your left ankle.

build up
Dragon Flow (page 46)

move forward
Golden Ball Warrior (page 96)

balance out
Seaweed Sway (page 106)

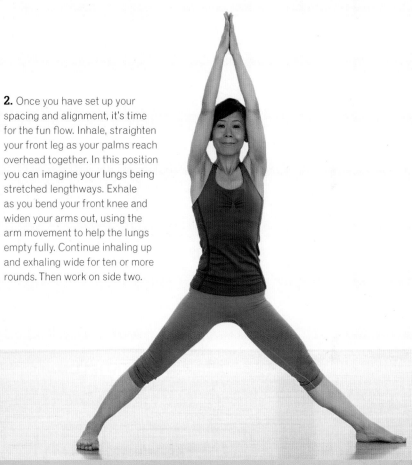

2. Once you have set up your spacing and alignment, it's time for the fun flow. Inhale, straighten your front leg as your palms reach overhead together. In this position you can imagine your lungs being stretched lengthways. Exhale as you bend your front knee and widen your arms out, using the arm movement to help the lungs empty fully. Continue inhaling up and exhaling wide for ten or more rounds. Then work on side two.

unwind
Quarter-Dog (page 60)

take care
Ensure that your knees mirror your toes in their direction of moment. The knee of the back leg will turn in slightly, just like the toes of the back leg.

☆ golden ball warrior

Influenced by qi gong, the arm movements of this pose support a
gathering-in of energy, to cup an imaginary golden ball of light and
then a soft and beautiful expansion outward. I use this a lot, because
I find it really helpful in bringing consciousness to the working of the
lungs. It works really well with Expansive Breath Warrior (see page 94).

1. Take a Warrior II position by stepping
your feet 1.2–1.5m (4–5ft) apart. Turn your
right leg and foot inward by 15 degrees.
Turn your left toes out by 90 degrees
and bend your left knee to sit it above
your left ankle. Ensure your left knee
doesn't sag inward, and that it stays
in line with the second toe.

Keep your right leg super-straight. Think
of lifting the inner arch of your right foot,
and feel a current of energy run up the
underside of the leg and thigh, creating
a lifting action. Take your arms to
horizontal, palms facing forward
so that your thumbs point up.

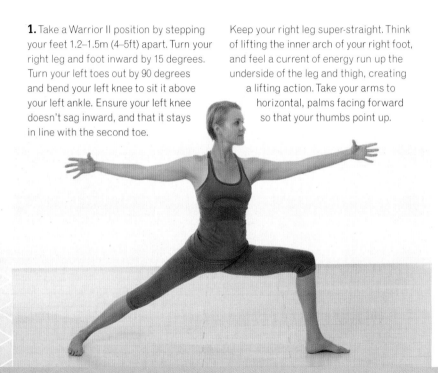

build up

Expansive Breath Warrior
(page 94)

move forward

Exultant Warrior Flow (page 98)

balance out

Seaweed Sway (page 106)

2. As you exhale, bend your elbows to float your palms closer together in front of your chest. Curl your fingers and soften your palms to cup an imaginary golden ball. Let your next inhalation carry your arms wide and back out to the side, as in step 1. Imagine the vacuum in your lungs, easily sucking in this fresh air so that your lungs broaden. Then exhale again and visualize your lungs narrowing as the elbows close in.

Continue for ten breaths or more. Enjoy the feeling of broadening and then narrowing your lungs, as the air moves in and out of them. Keep your legs working strongly so that your lower body position doesn't alter at all. Experience your base as strong and stable, while your torso, shoulders, arms and breath feel soft and floaty.

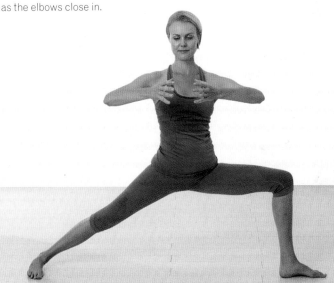

unwind
Kinky Cobbler's Pose (page 154)

take care
If you need an easier option, don't bend the front knee so far. Alternatively, straighten it completely with each inhalation.

☆ exultant warrior flow

This sequence becomes a graceful flow as each long, slow arm-sweep encourages a smooth, flowing breath. Bring awareness and constancy to the rate of air flow in and out, allowing the arm movements to be a mirror for the breath.

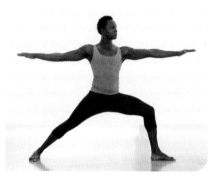 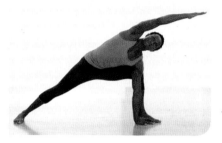

1. Stand with your legs wide apart. Go for about 1.3m (4½ft), or a little further if you are tall or have the flexibility. Turn your left foot out by 90 degrees and then, revolving from the right hip, allow the right leg and foot to turn in by 15 degrees. Bend your left knee to 90 degrees. Take your arms to horizontal. Look back to ensure your right shoulder isn't lifted, yet reinforce the muscular action along your back arm, so that it doesn't droop. Then settle your gaze on your left middle fingernail. This is your Warrior II pose.

2. To come into your Side-Angle Stretch, extend from your left hip to reach your left arm out and away. Bring your fingertips or flat palm to the floor near your left big toe. Press your left arm into your left leg, to help ease the knee backward a little, which will keep it tracking over your second toe. As you do this, take your right arm up and over, so that the upper arm sits just above your right ear, palm facing down. Create a strong line of energy by reaching from your right foot all the way to your right fingertips.

build up	**move forward**	**balance out**
Spine-Mobilizing Lunge (page 42)	Bound Side-Angle Stretch (see page 104)	Seaweed Sway (page 106)

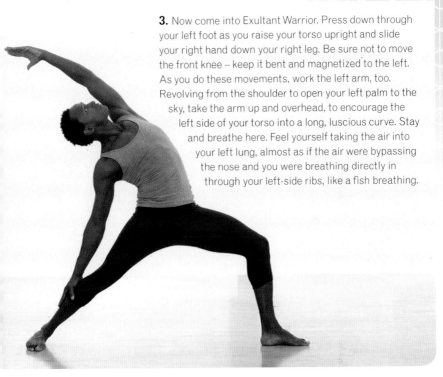

3. Now come into Exultant Warrior. Press down through your left foot as you raise your torso upright and slide your right hand down your right leg. Be sure not to move the front knee – keep it bent and magnetized to the left. As you do these movements, work the left arm, too. Revolving from the shoulder to open your left palm to the sky, take the arm up and overhead, to encourage the left side of your torso into a long, luscious curve. Stay and breathe here. Feel yourself taking the air into your left lung, almost as if the air were bypassing the nose and you were breathing directly in through your left-side ribs, like a fish breathing.

4. Now that your body has soaked up the correct alignment, you can speed things up to enjoy the flow. Inhale as your arms come to horizontal, returning to Warrior II as in step 1. Let the exhale take your reach out and down to Side-Angle Stretch as in step 2. On your next inhale, return to Warrior II, then exhale up and over to Exultant Warrior. After five or ten rounds, enjoy the second side.

unwind
Cow-Pose Spirals (page 222)

take care
Keep your front knee tracking correctly over the second toe below it. When you look down, you should be able to see your big toe, but not your smaller toes.

bowing side-angle pose

I love this pose, as it signifies courage in the face of vulnerability. To really bow your head low to the floor, you need to take your feet very wide apart. You must move mindfully and respect your body's limits, yet be fearless. This pose develops in us those excellent life skills of courage and determination.

STABLE AND STEADY: STANDING POSTURES

1. Start with your feet 1.2m (4ft) apart. Turn your left foot out by 90 degrees and turn your right leg and foot in by 15 degrees. Bend your left knee to sit directly above the left ankle. Rest your left elbow on your left thigh. Because the thrust of this movement will be to the left and forward, you need to develop a strong anchoring of your back leg. Look back at your right foot and press down through its little-toe edge. As you do this, lift the inner arch of the right foot slightly. You may experience a subtle lift of the inner knee and thigh away from the floor. Take your left foot wider and continue to ease your left knee forward, aiming to have it

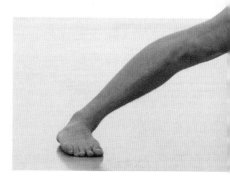

bent to 90 degrees. Once you have got your legs generously wide, bring in the shoulder action. Check that you feel safe and that your legs feel stable. There must be no sense of "losing" the grounding on the back foot or the lifting action along the back leg, because they provide a vital anchor.

build up
Bound Side-Angle Stretch
(see page 104)

move forward
Standing Splits (page 122)

balance out
Shoulder-Releasing Eagle
(page 116)

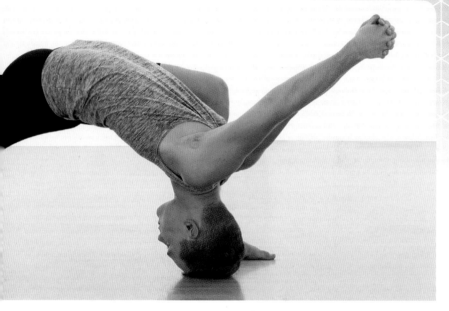

Interlace your fingers behind your back. Turn your belly and chest toward the ground and lower your whole torso to the floor. Bowing the head down, take your arms up and over. Let the reaching away with your knuckles lift your shoulders away from your ears. If you feel you want to take the legs wider, do so safely – take your fingertips to the floor first, to steady yourself. Reposition your legs, check that the back leg in particular is strongly rooted, then bring the arms back into your final pose.

unwind

Resting Pigeon (page 294)

take care

If you need greater stability and more help with balance, work with the legs closer together. Seek advice if you feel uncomfortable in your shoulders. Avoid inversions if you have high blood pressure, a risk of glaucoma or other eye issues, such as a detached retina.

☆ shoulder-stretching triangle

Not only will the fronts of your shoulders get a magnificent stretch in this pose, but you will find entering into the triangle shape with the arm positioned in this way gives you excellent alignment of the shoulders, hips and legs.

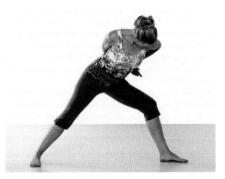 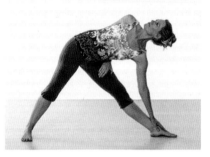

1. Start with your feet about 1.2m (4ft) apart. Turn your left knee and toes out by 90 degrees and your right thigh and foot inward by 15 degrees. Bring your left hand to your left knee. Tilt forward, letting your bottom move back. Take your right arm out to the right. Rotating from your shoulder, turn your right thumb down so that your palm faces back. Then slide the back of your hand across the lower back and hook the fingers to your left inner thigh. Grasp your right wrist with the left hand to help bring your hand lower. If you can't reach your thigh, hold the back of your waistband.

2. Once your fingers are hooked on, you can bring your posture into a pure alignment. Straighten your left knee as you move your hips forward and ease both shoulders backward. The two shoulders will line up over your left knee and ankle. While your left hip will be on the same plane as your left knee, do allow your right hip to be 5–7.5cm (2–3in) forward of the left. Choose a neck position that suits you, looking up, forward or down. Hold here and breathe. A small extra roll-back of the top shoulder can feel amazing.

build up	**move forward**	**balance out**
Yogic Clock (page 130)	Bound Side-Angle Stretch (see page 104)	Shoulder-Releasing Eagle (page 116)

3. Now release the arm and fly into a classic Triangle Pose. Keeping your legs and torso just where they were, extend your right arm to vertical and enjoy a new freedom in the shoulder. After several breaths, come out and practise side two.

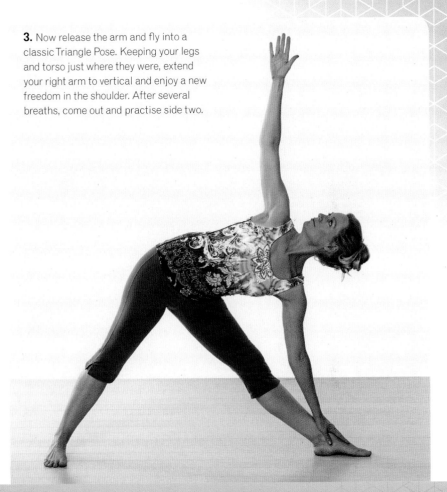

unwind
Corkscrew Twist (page 172)

take care
Don't push through any shoulder pain. Seek advice if you have a history of sacroiliac or shoulder issues.

bound side-angle stretch

The shoulder action in this pose really opens through the front of the shoulders, while the final straight-legged stage gives a deep stretch of the hamstring muscles. However, do remember that you don't have to reach the final stage of any pose to have a beautiful yoga practice. Yoga is about calming the mind, so practise being content with wherever your body gets to on any day.

1. Stand with your feet about 1.3–1.6m (4½–5¼ft) apart. Turn your left foot out by 90 degrees and turn your right thigh, knee and foot in by 15 degrees. Bend your left knee as close as you can get to 90 degrees. Take your left elbow to your left thigh. When you are ready, lean down to drop your left arm in front of your knee. Next, drop your shoulder even lower, to below the inner left knee. Now, rotate inward from the left shoulder and take your left hand under the left thigh.

Keep taking the hand back, reaching toward the sacrum. With the lower arm in position, reach your right arm up and rotate from the shoulder to turn the palm backward, thumb pointing down.

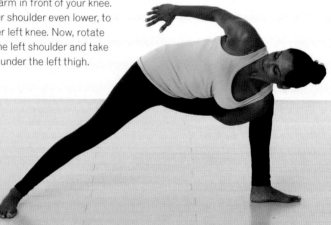

build up
Shoulder-Stretching Triangle
(page 102)

move forward
Bowing Side-Angle Pose
(page 100)

balance out
Seaweed Sway (page 106)

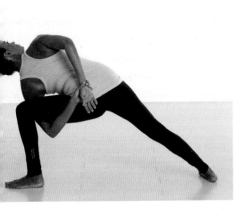

2. Now bend your right elbow and slide the back of the right hand across the lower back. If you can, curl the right and left fingertips together or, better still, hold your right wrist with your left hand. If you can't hold hands, grasp your clothing instead. Roll your top shoulder strongly back, then rotate your torso to the right and up. If that's comfortable for your neck, look up. If you are holding hands, try straightening both elbows and reaching your hands away, so that your hands are clear of your body. Create a steady breathing rhythm.

3. Move slowly to straighten your left leg for the amazing hamstring stretch. Deepen your pose by working again through the points in step 2. Hold for four to ten breaths before coming out, ready for the second side.

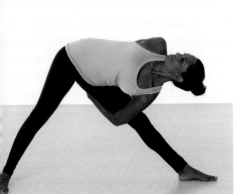

unwind
Three-Step Reclining Twist (page 170)

take care
Seek advice if you feel uncomfortable in the shoulders. When you are ready to straighten your front leg, do so very slowly so that you can monitor the release.

BOUND SIDE-ANGLE STRETCH

seaweed sway

How beautiful it is to learn to release deeply, even when you are technically standing. Once you get the true sense of the dangling relaxation this pose offers you, enjoy the way it feels as if even your brain releases. Let go of trying to control everything, and imagine your brain feeling delightfully slushy as you swish from side to side.

1. Stand with your legs wide apart. Position your feet so that their outer edges are parallel – your big toes will be closer together than your inner heels. Bend your knees and fold upside-down. If you have space, let your arms dangle, or if you are closer to the floor, fold your forearms to let them hang. You want everything from your hips down to your head, elbows and fingers to be soft and floppy. Check that your shoulders feel soft. Gently nod or a shake the head to release the neck. Stay in this position, and enjoy soft belly-breathing while you 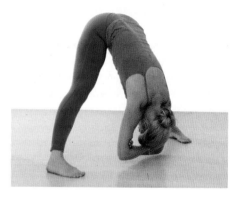 allow the weight of your head to ease your spine longer and flatter. This pose is about passively letting go and surrendering to gravity. If you don't feel you can open up to this sensation, bend your knees a lot more, which will help your torso to flatten, giving the sensation of sending your ribs through your inner thighs. This will help to create the feeling of dangling that you need in order to release and enjoy the pose. Visualize each of your vertebrae as a perfect pearl, strung together to form a beautiful long necklace.

build up	**move forward**	**balance out**
East–West Flow (page 48)	Deep Forward Bend at the Wall (page 152)	Flying Locust (page 38)

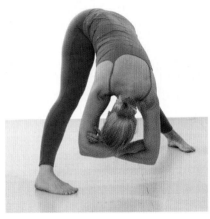

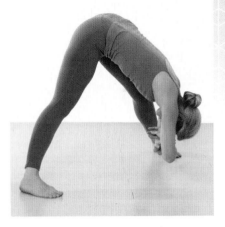

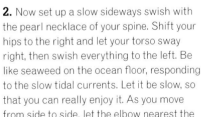

2. Now set up a slow sideways swish with the pearl necklace of your spine. Shift your hips to the right and let your torso sway right, then swish everything to the left. Be like seaweed on the ocean floor, responding to the slow tidal currents. Let it be slow, so that you can really enjoy it. As you move from side to side, let the elbow nearest the middle squeeze away from its hip and ease it closer to the floor. Enjoy the inner-thigh stretch as you sway. Continue to remind your neck muscles to let go, and allow the passive weight of your head, like a nice round coconut, to help the whole of your spine lengthen out.

unwind
Blissful Banana
(page 286)

take care
If you have a history of a slipped (herniated) disc in the lower back, keep your knees well bent and maintain an engaged core. Avoid forward bends completely if you have recent or active symptoms. Avoid inversions if you have high blood pressure, a risk of glaucoma or other eye issues, such as a detached retina.

shoulder-releasing forward fold

This pose is great for all body types, as you have a choice of where to place your emphasis. Once you are upside-down, you can choose whether you want to work the forward fold more by straightening the legs and lifting the sitting bones up. If you need to shoulder-release more, keep a deliberate bend in the knees so that your hamstrings don't draw your focus away from the deep shoulder release.

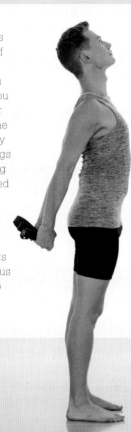

1. From standing, measure out your foot spacing by putting a fist between your big toes. This is the anatomical hip-width apart position for your feet. Take a yoga strap (or any soft belt, such as a bathrobe tie) and hold it between your hands behind your back. Hold the strap so that your hands are about 10cm (4in) apart. If you don't have a belt handy, interlace your fingers behind your back. Roll your shoulders back to broaden across your collar bones. Send a current of energy out through the arms and elbows as you reach your hands away from the shoulders, and then lift your hands as high up and far back as possible. Move your knuckles and chestbone away from each other.

build up
Shoulder Sweeps (page 34)

move forward
Flying Warrior (page 118)

balance out
Shoulder-Releasing Eagle (page 116)

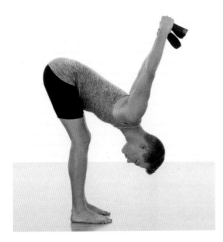

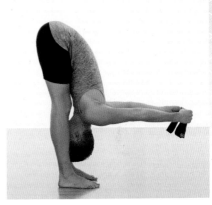

2. Fold forward from the hips. Choose whether you want your legs straight, to develop your hamstring stretch, or bent, so that you can focus on your shoulders. Once you are upside-down, continue to reach your hands away from your shoulders. If you are using a belt, pull on it, as if to separate your hands. You may feel a pleasant releasing sensation in the shoulders, as if you are making more space in the shoulder joints.

3. Now commence rolling first one shoulder forward, and then the other, as if you were practising freestyle swimming. After five or ten rolls, "swim" backstroke with each shoulder in turn. Enjoy the way the circular action softens the shoulders. Return to symmetry and again give a slow traction on the belt, to work deeper into the shoulders. Then bend the knees and stand up, and feel your shoulders smile at you.

unwind
Twisty Tree (page 114)

take care
Seek professional advice on which movements are suitable if you have a shoulder injury. Avoid forward bends if you are at risk of disc injury. Avoid inversions if you have high blood pressure, a risk of glaucoma or other eye issues, such as a detached retina.

revolved half-moon flow

This lovely sequence will develop your skill in balancing, plus build flexibility in forward folding, as you move mindfully through three classic yoga poses: taking Intense Forward Stretch through Revolved Triangle Pose and into the Revolved Half-Moon Flow.

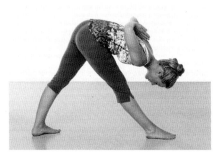

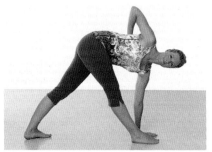

1. With your right leg in front, stand with your feet 1m (3¼ft) apart. While your front foot points forward, have your back foot turned out by 15 degrees. Square your hips to the front and take your arms out wide. Roll the shoulders forward as you turn your thumbs down and bend the elbows, to bring the palms together behind your back. Wiggle your palms higher up your back. Revolve your abdomen to the right a little, then fold from the hips into Intense Forward Stretch. Anchor through the back foot and move your right hip forward. Hold for five breaths.

2. Flow into Revolved Triangle Pose. Leave your right hand in position and take your left hand to the floor, by the big toe. If you need to, bend your knee to reduce any rounding of the spine. That lovely long feeling through your spine will improve your twisting action. It's nice to press the left hand into your back, to "push" you into the twist. Stack your shoulders by moving your left shoulder to the right and your right shoulder up and back. If you can, move your left hand to the little-toe edge of the foot. If it's comfortable, look up. Breathe for five long breaths.

build up	**move forward**	**balance out**
Dragon Flow (page 46)	Sage Pose with Neck Releases (page 176)	Cobbler's Bridge (page 192)

3. Now move into Revolved Half-Moon Flow. Look down and move your left hand about 30cm (12in) forward and a little to the right of the big toe. Take a small step forward with your back foot, coming onto the back toes. Lift your back leg up to horizontal. Lower your right hip, yet maintain a strong lift with the left thigh and knee, to prevent the foot drooping lower than the hip. Now "free" your right arm by flying it up to vertical. Further develop the twist in the torso, and again aim to stack the shoulders by moving the left shoulder further to the right and the right shoulder to the left. Hold for five breaths. Then move through the Classic Downward-Facing Dog Pose (see page 58) and practise side two.

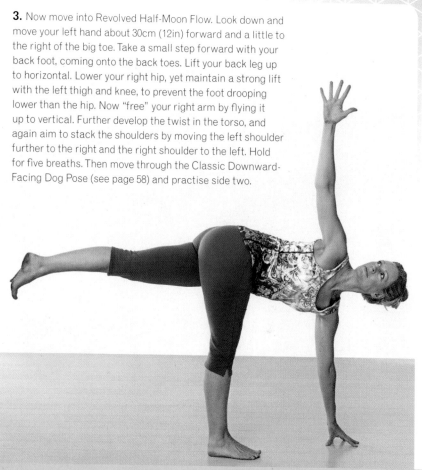

unwind
East–West Flow (page 48)

take care
Be careful of these twisting and forward-bending postures if you have a history of disc herniation. Avoid inversions if you have high blood pressure, a risk of glaucoma or other eye issues, such as a detached retina.

REVOLVED HALF-MOON FLOW

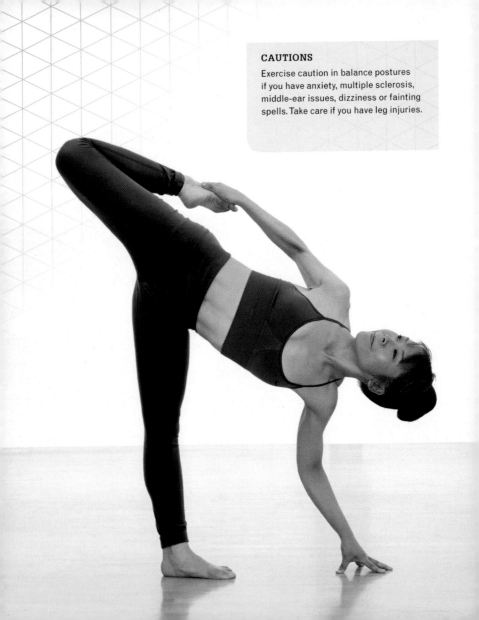

5.

BALANCING BALMS

Balancing postures tone. They stretch, they strengthen. But when my students ask for them in class, it's usually because they want to calm a scattered mind. It's simple: the more speedily we race through our modern lives, the more we crave those moments where we stop, stand still and take stock. Finding your bodily balance spills over to the psycho-emotional realm, too – a balance pose can feel as if it's bringing you closer to your calm centre. Balances naturally draw the wandering mind inward. And the focus required to balance relieves stress, as you need to mentally return to the present moment.

A bit of balance-prowess makes injuries from falling later in life less likely, so these postures are yoga life insurance for the years ahead. You can relax, smiling, into those little wobbles, knowing that your nervous and muscular systems are masterfully fine-tuning with your adjustments and micro-adjustments. You will experience how any tiny alteration in a single part of your body will mean that all the other parts subtly shift to accommodate this change. This creates a beautiful sense of harmony throughout your whole body, and you will learn to trust it more through balance postures.

Life just feels better when we are fluid and stable, so enjoy developing these patterns in finding your balance on the mat, and in balancing your life off the mat.

☆ twisty tree

Bringing movement into any one-legged posture always increases the challenge. Visualize your bones stacking in perfect alignment, and trust that your muscles need only do the minimum to hold you tall. Then all the hard work melts away and you can get on with enjoying your shape and your breath.

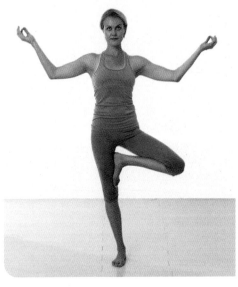

1. Come into your basic Tree Pose: from standing, ground down through the right foot and bend your left knee up. Take hold of your left ankle, and position your foot as high up your right inner thigh as possible while avoiding the knee joint. The lower the foot is, the easier it is to balance. Press the sole of your foot against your inner thigh, while at the same time resisting back with the inner thigh toward the sole of the foot. This will keep you feeling more stable. Touch your thumbs to your index fingers and take your arms up to the sides, elbows bent and palms facing up.

build up
Spine Mobilizer (page 50)

move forward
Standing Splits (page 122)

balance out
Seaweed Sway (page 106)

BALANCING BALMS

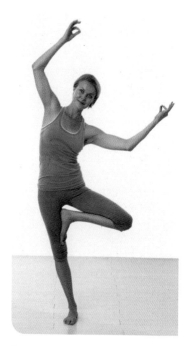

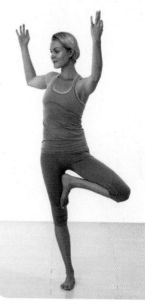

3. Come upright and make your Twisty Tree. First twist to your right, away from your bent knee. Firm your abdominal muscles to help you revolve as deeply as

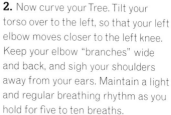

2. Now curve your Tree. Tilt your torso over to the left, so that your left elbow moves closer to the left knee. Keep your elbow "branches" wide and back, and sigh your shoulders away from your ears. Maintain a light and regular breathing rhythm as you hold for five to ten breaths.

possible. Notice how your breathing changes. After several breaths, return to the centre and revolve to your left. This might feel more satisfying, as you can go further. Again, it's your core muscles that will pull you around most obviously, but do appreciate the working of the back muscles, too. After several breaths, return to the centre. Come back onto two feet, re-centre and practise side two.

unwind
Three-Step Shoulder Release (page 52)

take care
Wedge your bent knee to a wall if you are worried about toppling over. Seek advice before practising one-legged poses if you suffer from vertigo or dizzy spells.

shoulder-releasing eagle

In this modern take on the Eagle, your lower body will work extra-hard to stay stable despite the challenge of the upper-body movements. I like it, as it feels like tricking your tight shoulders into softening as they respond to the flowing movements of your arms. It's about having an undemanding attitude to these gentler gliding stretches, which avoid the harsh demands of a long hold.

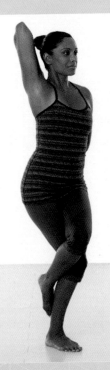

1. From standing, bend both knees. Lift your left knee up and take it across your right thigh. If you can, wrap your leg all the way around, so that your left ankle locks behind your right calf. If that movement isn't possible for you, take your left ankle to your right thigh, just near the knee. Once you have found your leg position, bend your standing leg deeply and tilt forward from the hips, to get more release in the gluteal muscles. Extend your arms out wide and begin to travel your left arm down and your right arm up. As you come toward vertical with each arm, bend the elbows to bring your hands together behind your back. Hook the fingers together. If your hands can't reach each other, get as close as you can for today – time and practice will take care of that, so smile that you are here now, patiently enjoying the journey as tensions dissolve.

build up
Half-Reverse Prayer (page 138)

move forward
Pyramid Prayer (page 140)

balance out
Three-Up Bridge Pose
(page 246)

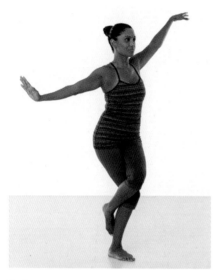
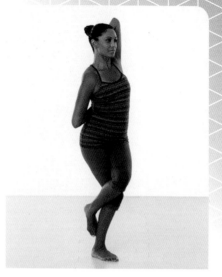

2. Once this movement is complete, switch your arms to the second side. Release your finger grasp, and straighten both elbows. Inhale to circle both arms long and wide, as your left arm floats up while your right arm sinks. Exhale as both elbows bend and the fingers reclaim their grasp. Don't be surprised if one side feels stiffer than the other – I tell my students it just means they are a human being who has lived. Accept your asymmetries, smile kindly upon yourself and keep practising.

3. Stay balancing on one leg as you continue to move in time with your breath. Inhale as you circle to reach your arms vertically up and down, then exhale to bend and clasp. Set up a slow flow, alternating from side to side, while your shoulders soften in their acceptance of the stretches. After about eight rounds, come back to standing on two feet. Take some time to note where your body has released.

unwind
Hip-Releasing Wide Child Pose
(page 216)

take care
Get clearance from an expert if you have shoulder issues.
Seek advice before practising one-legged poses if you suffer
from vertigo or dizzy spells.

flying warrior

You'll find strength you didn't know you possessed as you practise this pose. It demands a real commitment, to go all the way upside-down and stay there. Use your warrior-like courage to develop your mastery while you remain steady and focused.

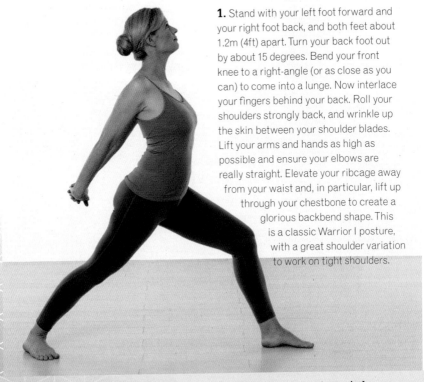

1. Stand with your left foot forward and your right foot back, and both feet about 1.2m (4ft) apart. Turn your back foot out by about 15 degrees. Bend your front knee to a right-angle (or as close as you can) to come into a lunge. Now interlace your fingers behind your back. Roll your shoulders strongly back, and wrinkle up the skin between your shoulder blades. Lift your arms and hands as high as possible and ensure your elbows are really straight. Elevate your ribcage away from your waist and, in particular, lift up through your chestbone to create a glorious backbend shape. This is a classic Warrior I posture, with a great shoulder variation to work on tight shoulders.

build up
Standing Splits
(page 122)

move forward
Dancer's Bow
(page 124)

balance out
Cow-Pose Spirals
(page 222)

unwind
Reclining Eagle Twist
(page 226)

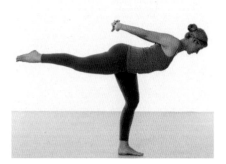

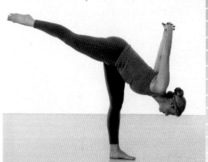

2. Take a small step forward with your back foot, coming up to tiptoes. Lean your torso forward slightly, so that you come out of the backbend. Contract your abdominal muscles, creating a muscular connection between your lowest ribs in front and your hip bones. This will help enormously during your one-legged balancing. Tilt forward some more, as you lift your back leg all the way up to horizontal. Your right hip will probably have lifted, compared to your left, so drop it down so that you are flat across your sacrum. In Flying Warrior, continue to reach your knuckles away with energy to stretch the fronts of both shoulders.

3. If you can, take this pose upside-down. Squeeze on your abdominals and, lengthening out from the tailbone, tilt forward at the hips. If you don't travel far, bend your standing leg to go further. On your flying leg, squeeze on the muscles of the front thigh to reach it further up and away. Fan out the toes of the right foot. Reach your arms up and over as far as they will go. Be like a bicycle wheel – from the centre of your pelvis, radiate your "spokes" out and away strongly in three directions: up and over with the arms, grounding down with the standing leg, and up and away with the flying leg. Stay for five breaths and then, with control, return to step 1. Bring your feet together and change sides.

take care

It's always possible to practise one-legged standing poses on two legs while you develop your balancing skills. Keep your back big toe on the floor to help, while still focusing your weight-bearing on the front leg. Avoid inversions during menstruation and if you have eye issues, such as a detached retina or a risk of glaucoma. Seek advice before practising one-legged poses if you suffer from vertigo or dizzy spells.

sugar-cane goddess pose

A backbend, a twist, a forward bend and a balance – this multifaceted posture yields many fruits. It will give you strength, stability and flexibility, while the balance element encourages the mind to quieten. Then all your good efforts will be yoked together for an overall focusing effect.

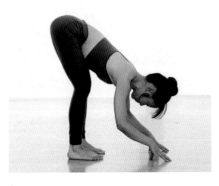 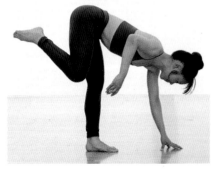

1. Start with your feet hip-width apart. Fold forward and bend the knees enough to enable your ribs to drop closer to your thighs, so that your vertebral column feels as if it is dangling. With your fingertips to the floor, release the neck and shoulder muscles to allow the head to hang, pleasantly heavy. Relax into this for several long breaths, letting gravity do its work.

2. Next, transfer your weight onto your left foot and left hand. Start to lift your right leg and arm up and out to the side. Keep these two limbs soft, to create a sense of unfurling as you open up and out to the side.

build up
Gate Pose with Side Bow (page 44)

move forward
Dancer's Bow (page 124)

balance out
Standing Splits (page 122)

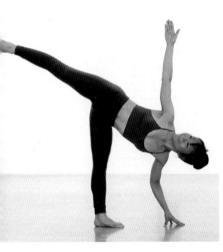 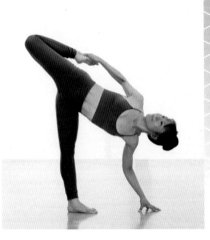

3. Now come into a classic Half-Moon Pose. Float your right arm and straighten it, reaching it up to vertical. Then press your right heel away, pressing actively through your right leg and foot. Straighten your standing leg as much as your inner-thigh flexibility will allow. Some people enjoy making a T-shape, with their torso and leg on a horizontal plane. Others like to lift the right leg higher, to allow the torso to drop down, as shown. Stay there for five breaths.

4. To transition to Sugar-Cane Goddess Pose, bend your right knee in toward your abdomen. Catch your foot with your right hand. Then open through the front of the hip and send the knee back and away. Press your right heel to your right buttock. Anchoring through your left fingertips, rotate your torso to the right and upward. Moving from your belly will create a spiralling sensation. After five to ten breaths, return to the soft forward fold (step 1), and then practise side two.

unwind
Half-and-Half Dog (page 61)

take care
If your neck feels really good, tuck your chin in slightly and look up to the sky; otherwise, look out horizontally or turn your face down, as required. Avoid inversions if you have high blood pressure, a risk of glaucoma or other eye issues, such as a detached retina.

standing splits

This pose certainly looks like the super-stretchy hamstring release it is. But what I really love about it is a bit unexpected. Like a secret gift bestowed with a whisper, its surprise is how deep the stretch-out for the lower back is. Try it out and see how it makes you feel.

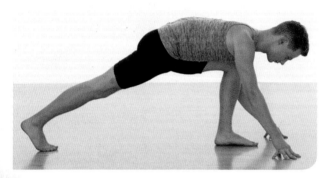

Bend your left knee again and move your right fingertips about 30cm (12in) in front of your big toe, keeping your hand to the right of the foot. Wrap your left forearm against your left calf, elbow bent, so that your forearm is vertical and your hand wraps above the heel. Take a small step in with the back foot and come onto your right toes, ready for lift-off.

1. Start with your legs wide apart with your left foot in front. Turn your left foot out to 45 degrees and turn your right leg and foot in a little. Fold over to bring your fingers to the floor. Walk your fingertips to your left, bringing one hand on each side of the foot. Bend into your left knee and come up onto your fingertips, to give the torso clearance for the next move. As you inhale first lift the chest up, then twist your belly strongly to the left, to line up your chestbone with your left thigh bone. Then, when you exhale, you can lay your chest on your thigh, possibly straightening that leg to warm up for the stronger hamstring stretch that is coming.

build up
Tension-Releasing Forward Fold (page 156)

move forward
Intense Reclining Side-Stretch (page 196)

balance out
Cobbler's Bridge (page 192)

BALANCING BALMS

2. Transfer your weight to your left foot and lift up the right leg. Press the leg up and away, while you balance on your left leg and right hand. Now seek to close the gap between your torso and left thigh. If possible, straighten your standing leg. Increase the challenge by walking your right fingertips back to come level with your left toes. Ensure both legs are super-straight and send that flying leg up to vertical. Squeeze the muscles of the front thigh, to help lift it even more. If you can, instead of looking down, untuck your chin and look across on the horizontal. Keep working to "glue" your belly and chest to your thigh. And last but not least, breathe! After five or more breaths, come down lightly and with control. Walk your hands across to the right and adjust your feet, ready for side two.

3. If you really want to go for it, with an increased twisting action plus a strong shoulder stretch, change the arm position in step 2. Wrap your right arm on the outside of your left leg, by crossing your right shoulder over the front of the left shin.

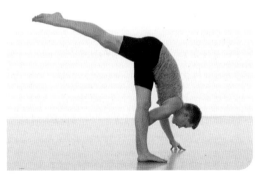

STANDING SPLITS

---

unwind
Backbend Ripple (page 290)

take care
Ensure that your hamstrings are warmed up before you begin by completing a few forward bends.

dancer's bow

Many standing balances are fairly static postures. This Dancer's Bow starts off as a classic yoga *asana*, and then a bit of fun comes in when you try to take it upside-down. With the strong hamstring stretch, it's a forward bend within a backbend. And due to the one-legged movement, it's harder than it looks to balance. Try it out and have fun.

1. From standing, extend your right leg back, touching your toes to the floor behind you. Square your hips to the front. Bend the right knee, and reach back with your right hand to catch the foot. Notice how your ribcage has lost its symmetry, and reinforce the forward propulsion through the right side to square it off with the left as much as possible. As you reach the right foot up and back to create your Dancer's pose, tip your torso forward. Reach your left arm out in front, palm up. Place the tips of your thumb and index-finger together. Each time you practise Dancer's Bow you can alternate between having your standing leg bent or, as shown, straight. Remind yourself that good balancing doesn't mean holding a shape perfectly still. Invite in the tiny movements and micro-adjustments as you find and refine your centre. Hold for five breaths.

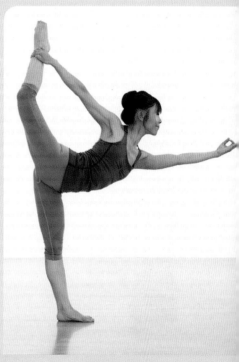

build up
Gate Pose with Side Bow
(page 44)

move forward
Bow Pose Three Ways
(page 238)

balance out
Revolved Happy Pose
(page 174)

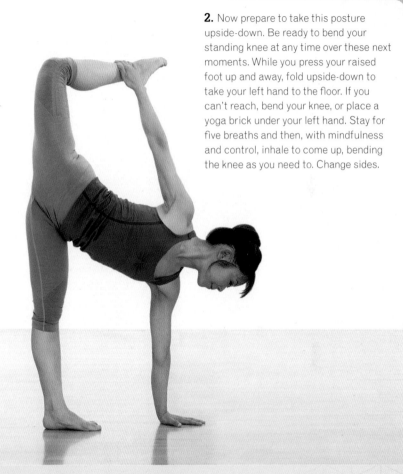

2. Now prepare to take this posture upside-down. Be ready to bend your standing knee at any time over these next moments. While you press your raised foot up and away, fold upside-down to take your left hand to the floor. If you can't reach, bend your knee, or place a yoga brick under your left hand. Stay for five breaths and then, with mindfulness and control, inhale to come up, bending the knee as you need to. Change sides.

unwind
Banana Pose (page 194)

take care

If you are concerned about falling, work within reach of a stable chair, table or wall. Avoid inversions if you have eye issues such as a detached retina or a risk of glaucoma.

big-toe balance

This pose will develop concentration and poise. Any balance pose will offer you an invitation to equilibrium, so while strength is certainly required to move in and out of the *asana*, you'll also enjoy the calm and tranquil aspects of this posture.

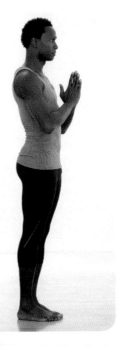

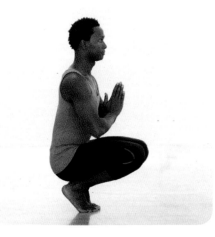

1. Stand with your feet together in Mountain Pose. Bring your palms together at your heart centre in the middle of your chest. Enjoy the length in your spine and notice its natural curves.

2. Lift up onto tiptoe and feel your abdominal muscles activate. As you prepare to bend your knees and lower down, do your best to resist the urge to tilt the torso forward. Instead, as you lower your hips to your lifted heels in a low squat, move as if you were in an elevator, keeping your spine as vertical as possible.

build up
Head-Beyond-the-Knee Pose (page 160)

move forward
Power Squat (page 218)

balance out
Locust Sway (page 234)

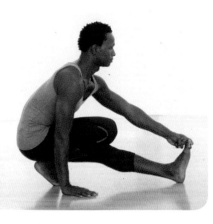

3. Place your hands to the floor to steady yourself and extend your left leg straight out, heel to the floor. Lean forward and then reach out your left hand to loop your big toe with your first two fingers. If you can't reach, grasp a soft belt looped around the ball of the foot.

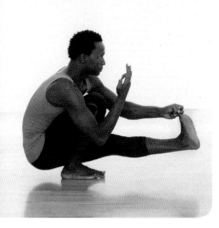

4. Lift your left leg in the air as you counterbalance by dropping the right heel down to the floor. Bring your torso to an upright position and activate the muscles of your whole back. Squeezing on the muscles of the upper back will uncurve the spine, so you can then lift as tall as possible. Hold your right hand in a classic yoga hand-gesture called Jnana Mudra, with the tips of thumb and index finger touching. Allow the elbow to bend down and the palm to face up. Stay there for five to ten breaths. Then release your foot and slide it back in, so the feet come together. With your palms together, lift your hips to come up to Mountain Pose, then lift back up onto tiptoes, ready for the other side.

BIG-TOE BALANCE

unwind
Restorative Twist (page 292)

take care
Avoid this pose and seek further advice
if you experience knee pain.

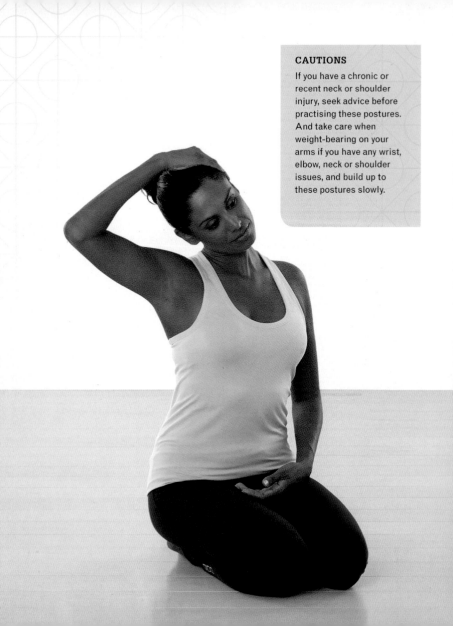

6.

STRONG NECK, STRETCHY SHOULDERS

Two things most commonly requested by students in a yoga class are relief for a tight neck and quality shoulder-openers. In this section you will find both, and there are more such exercises scattered throughout the book. Some of these postures link the whole body, and others you can bring into your day *off* the mat –

poses that you can practise at your desk and sneak into those spare moments.

So if you find that your neck and shoulders seem to be a reservoir for stress, make peace with those tight muscles and give your neck and shoulders the yoga-love they have been craving.

☆ yogic clock

A spring-clean for the shoulders, this sequence erases shoulder tension. And, best of all, you can do it just about anywhere: use a wall in your home or office, get creative at the bus stop or find a friendly tree.

1. Stand side-on to the wall, with the wall to your left. Position your left foot about 15cm (6in) from the wall. Have your feet hip-width apart, with both sets of toes pointing straight ahead. Get the maximum stretch possible by coming up onto tiptoes to take your left palm as high up the wall as possible. With your palm pressed firmly to the wall, over several long exhalations, slowly lower your heels to the floor. Imagine your left palm is glued to the wall and resist sliding it down while you lower your heels. Trust in the releasing ability of your exhalations to allow the soft tissues of your whole body to lengthen, so that you can do your best stretch through your shoulder and down your torso. Now add in a stretch for the left side of your neck. Lightly tuck in your chin and revolve your head to look down the front of your right shoulder. Hinge your right wrist, to press out through the heel of that hand. As you do this, aim to keep each hip sitting over each ankle below, so that you resist leaning toward the wall. After several breaths here, return your head and neck to a forward-looking position.

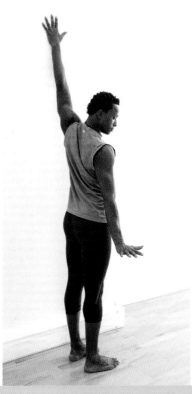

build up	**move forward**	**balance out**
Shoulder Sweeps (page 34)	Cow-Pose Spirals (page 222)	Eagle Shoulder Stretch (page 132)

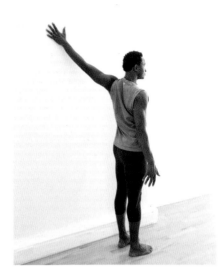
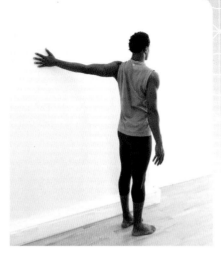

2. From the vertical left-arm position, like 12 o'clock, move your left arm back a few notches, to half-past ten on your imaginary clock face. Stretch the skin and fingers of your left hand and reach it as far back as possible. Without moving your left hand at all, lean your body forward, to increase the shoulder and chest-muscle stretch. Stay here for eight or more breaths, allowing the front of your shoulder to release deeply.

3. Finally, move your hand to half-past nine on the clock. With palm glued to the wall, lean your torso forward as you enjoy this effective release for the shoulders. After eight or more breaths, come out and let both arms hang by your sides. Notice how thoroughly different your two shoulders feel. Most likely the one you have stretched will feel warm, loose, vibrant and alive. Your other shoulder deserves to feel this good, too, so turn around and work with the second side using the clock positions of 12 o'clock, half-past two and half-past three.

unwind
Quarter-Dog (page 60)

take care
If you have an injury or experience any shoulder pain, seek advice from an expert before continuing.

☆ eagle shoulder stretch

Take the classic Eagle arm position, add a pinch of Mountain Pose and
stir it up with a bit of flow: what a great recipe for healthy shoulders!
By releasing any build-up of tension between the shoulder blades,
these flowing movements will help bring a smile back to sad shoulders.

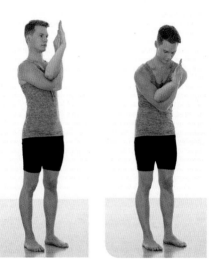

1. Stand with
your feet hip-
width apart.
Spread both
arms out wide,
then bring
them toward
each other in
front. As they come together in front, drop
your right elbow down and slip it across,
up and around to the left of your left upper
arm. Then, if you can manage it, cross
over at the forearms as well, to bring the
right fingers to touch the left palm.

2. Keeping your arms intertwined, draw circles
with your elbows. Move in a clockwise direction.
Go as wide as you can to each side, and get
plenty of height for your circle, too. Allow your
shoulders to dance a little, and notice how your
torso twists to respond to the movement.

build up	**move forward**	**balance out**
Circle of Joy (page 30)	Half-Reverse Prayer (page 138)	Yin Child with a Twist (page 315)

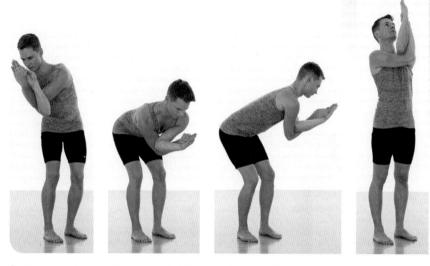

3. Once your shoulders have accepted the stretch, expand the movement out to involve your whole torso. Tip forward from the hips and circle your entire body in a clockwise direction as well.

4. After five rounds of these big circles, come back to standing tall. Unravel your arms and let them dangle. Take time to note where your body has released. Then inhale to widen your arms to horizontal. Exhale and entwine them again, this time with the left arm under the right. Circle anticlockwise, before adding in the larger movements of the torso.

unwind
Blissful Banana (page 286)

take care
Engage your abdominals and bend your knees a little to protect your back as you make your large circles.

☆ seated neck stretch and strengthen

Develop an even steadiness in the muscles that support the neck to keep it feeling well aligned. The key is to take short holds while you learn how your neck responds. Neck stretches are a bit like medicine – a little is good for you, but you don't want to take too much.

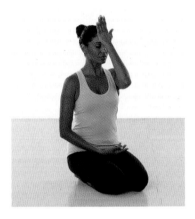

1. Sit or kneel in any comfortable position that allows your spine to feel tall. Imagine you have a ripe peach between your chin and chest. Most likely your chin will tuck in, but don't overdo it and bruise the fruit – you want to enjoy the natural inward curve of your neck. Take one palm to your forehead. Set up a light pressure of your forehead against it. Resist with your palm just enough to ensure that you don't travel anywhere. Hold for three breaths, before resting and repeating.

2. Now interlace both hands behind your head. Again, ensure you maintain the natural curve of those precious neck vertebrae, but drop the chin down subtly, which will activate some important stabilizers – the deep neck flexor muscles. Press your head back into your hands, while resisting with the hands so that no outward movement occurs. Hold for three breaths. Rest and repeat. Then, with a light pressure from the hands, drop your chin to your throat for a gentle neck stretch, over three or four breaths.

build up	**move forward**	**balance out**
Circle of Joy (page 30)	Sage Pose with Neck Releases (page 176)	Tiger Flow (page 32)

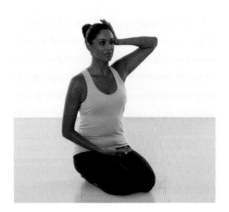

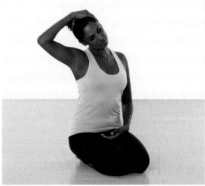

3. Now do the same for the muscles on the side of the neck. Place one palm against your ear. With your head in a neutral position, press your head and palm against each other while staying still. After three breaths, rest and repeat. Then move on to side two.

4. Finally, combine a lateral neck stretch with some strength work. Tilt your head to the right and reach your right arm up overhead, to place your right fingers over your left ear. Press down with your palm, yet resist upward with your head for three breaths. Then let go of the resistance, as the light palm pressure offers you a stretch all the way down the side of the neck to the tip of the left shoulder. After three breaths, lower your arm and bring your head upright, ready for side two.

unwind
Eagle Shoulder Stretch (page 132)

take care
Seek advice before practising this pose if you have neck issues. Use a light pressure only and don't stay in it for too long.

magical shoulder and neck release

You will feel so good after this neat little exercise that the only word for it is…magical.

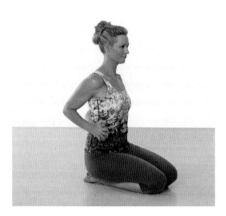 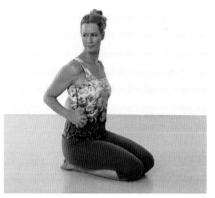

1. Kneel in the Hero Pose, as shown, or take any seated position where your spine can float tall. Take both arms behind your back. Interlace your fingers, and then pull both hands around to the right side of your waist. Take a few mindful, yet firm pulls, to ease both sets of knuckles forward. You may be able to draw both hands to the front of your body. If possible, close both wrists toward each other. Ensure your torso doesn't twist off to one side, and keep it facing square-on to the front. Do your best to maintain a neutral spine position, too, resisting the tendency to move into a backbend shape. Now roll both shoulders back and squeeze your elbows toward each other. Stay here for five to ten breaths.

2. For the next step, add in a neat little neck release. Turn your head to look to the right. Draw your chin toward your throat so that your eyes will look down, then release it so that your eyes look out horizontal again. Set up a nodding action by repeating the chin tuck-and-release a few more times. Then return your head to centre, and bring your arms to your sides. Notice any changes that have occurred in your neck and shoulders. Then repeat on the second side.

☆ playful shoulder release

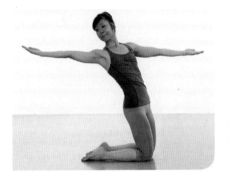

I've named this pose to inspire you to go back in time and find that playful inner child that resides within you. These moves feel as if they make the brain think in a slightly different way and help us lighten up. Find the sense of joy and fun, as you make your shoulders happy.

1. In a high kneeling position, reach both arms overhead. Tuck your tailbone under to bring your hips into a posterior tilt position. Exhale as you lean back, enjoying a front thigh stretch and a bit of core-strengthening. Inhale as you return to vertical. Flow together your backward and forward movements and breaths a few more times.

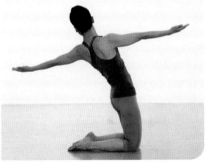

2. The next time you lean back, reach your right arm back while you take your left arm forward. Circle the arms, so that both reach downward as you are at your deepest lean backward. As both arms complete their circles to reach up overhead, your body returns to vertical. Continue for five or more rounds with the arms circling in this direction.

3. The next time both arms meet overhead, change directions to circle your arms the opposite way. As you complete five or more rounds, remind yourself that you are doing this to soften your tight shoulders. So soften your brain a little, too. Sometimes we over-think things. Remove all that mental tension of trying too hard – just relax and have fun.

half-reverse prayer

This is a great stretch for anyone who spends long hours at a desk, or for parents who carry small children. You will always have a tighter side, but remember: you don't need to attach any blame or judgement to that – it's not helpful to the opening process. Instead, send your tighter side a little more loving energy. Developing a kind, healing attention will allow your tight spots to open in their own time.

1. Sit on the floor with your legs bent up in front of you. Take your left arm out to the side and, rotating from the shoulder, turn the palm to the back so the thumb points down. Bend your elbow and slide the back of your hand up your back. Cup your left elbow with your right hand and ease the elbow toward the midline of your body. As you do this, snuggle your left fingers up your back, as if they were trying to tickle the back of your neck.

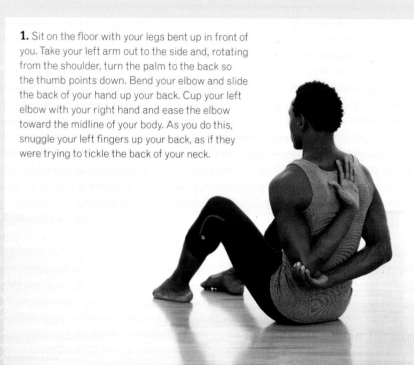

build up
Shoulder-Loving Cobra
(page 230)

move forward
Crocodile Build-Up (page 144)

balance out
Playful Shoulder Release
(page 137)

STRONG NECK, STRETCHY SHOULDERS

2. Once you have drawn your left elbow in as much as possible, hold it in place and lie yourself down on the floor. Choose your most-relaxed leg position: you can bend your knees up or lengthen them out along the floor. Rest your right arm on the floor. Now use your breathing to get deeper into the stretch. Inhale light and warmth into your shoulder, and exhale away any tensions. If you sense that your shoulder can go one step further, roll your left shoulder back to increase the sensation. Stay here for one or two minutes. Roll to the right side to come out and sit up. When you practise the second side, remember that while your body may have tightened up in response to life's impacts, it is doing the very best it can for you. Be grateful for all its good efforts.

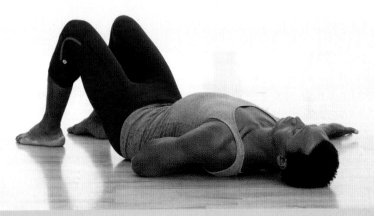

unwind
Shoulder Sweeps (page 34)

take care
If you experience any shoulder or neck pain, seek advice from an expert before continuing.

pyramid prayer

While this pose focuses on the shoulders, the whole back and legs get a great stretch, too. It's a fabulous one to do when you feel that mid-afternoon energy dip. I love seeing how the look in my students' eyes has changed. You can see that many have found a deep relaxation, as they come up after a nice long hold in this pose.

1. Stand facing a table or similar support. Your right foot should be about 30cm (12in) from the support, toes pointing forward. Step your left leg back about 60cm (2ft) and turn your foot out by 15 degrees. Bend your front knee and fold forward to place your elbows on the support, shoulder-width apart. Then bring your palms together with fingers pointing upward. Ease your hips back, so that your back comes to a flat shape. Position your head so that your ears are between your upper arms. The more you can move your hips back and create that long, flat feeling in your spine, the easier it will be for your head to clear the ledge. If you can, straighten your front knee and deepen the crease where your right thigh joins your torso. This will allow your right hip to move backward a little, which will keep the hips square. Stay here for eight or more breaths.

2. If you would like to add to this stretch, bend both elbows and take your thumbs to the spine between your shoulder blades. Do this on an exhalation, then inhale to return your forearms up to a vertical position. Repeat a few more times, exhaling down, then inhaling back up. Step forward to come up. Then repeat with your left leg in front.

build up
Quarter-Dog (page 60)

move forward
Forearm Balance (page 276)

balance out
Dancer's Bow (page 124)

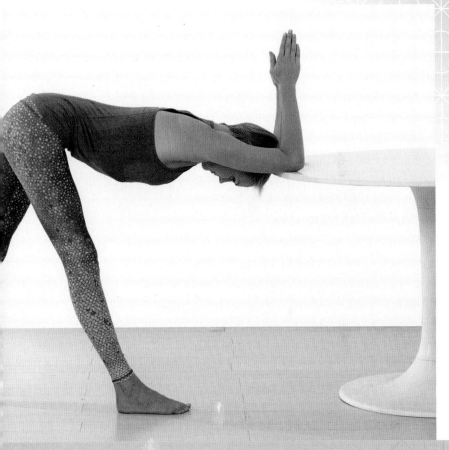

unwind
Seaweed Sway (page 106)

take care
If you experience any shoulder or neck pain,
seek advice from an expert before continuing.

slinky shoulders, gleeful glutes

I teach this one *a lot*, because people need it *a lot*. It's a combination of two classic poses: it adopts the lower-body position of Cow Face Pose, and the upper-body position of Eagle Pose. It feels as if it gets rid of the dust and the rust, allowing your body to move lightly and freely.

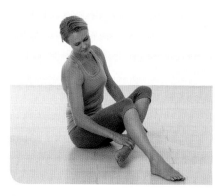

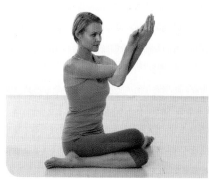

1. Sit on the floor with your legs bent up in front. Take your right arm underneath your right thigh to grasp your left ankle. Pull your left foot through, to rest on the floor by your right hip. Position your left knee to the midline of your body, as much as possible. Now take your right ankle in your left hand. Lift the leg up and over to the left, so that your right foot rests by your left outer hip. As much as your hips will allow, stack your right knee on top of your left.

2. Open your arms wide and bring them together, dropping your left elbow under the right one to interlock your upper arms. Entwine them again at the forearms or wrists, so that your palms face each other.

build up
Shoulder Sweeps (page 34)

move forward
Twisted Pigeon (page 182)

balance out
Hip-Releasing Wide Child Pose (page 216)

3. Set up a contraction that will work deeply into the back of the shoulders. Squeeze your right elbow to the right, and resist as you squeeze your left elbow to the left. As the resistance is equal, you won't travel anywhere. Hold for several breaths.

Now do the same sort of thing, only up and down. Press your top elbow down while pushing up with your lower elbow for several breaths. Again, with even resistance, you won't move outwardly, but you may well feel a good release in the shoulders. Repeat the horizontal and vertical pressure-squeezes, if you like. Finally, let go of the contraction work. Lift both elbows higher and straighten them as much as you can, without losing the upper-arm lock. Mentally direct your breath into the space between your shoulder blades to help this area soften and open. Add in a forward fold to awaken the hips. If you are flexible, aim your elbows beyond your knees. Breathe for five to ten slow breaths. Then come out and practise side two.

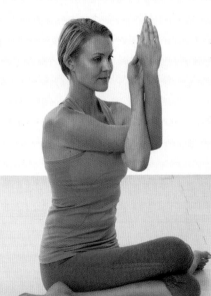

unwind
Banana Pose (page 194)

take care
If you can't get your knees close to stacking, try lengthening the lower leg out straight, so that only the top leg is bent. If that's not possible, take an easy cross-legged pose instead.

crocodile build-up and crocodile

Lifting one leg up and back, like the tail of a tiger, is such a great way to take the edge off while you develop the strength needed to safely practise the yoga Plank and Crocodile Poses. These are important poses to master, because they often feature in modern yoga's more flowing practices.

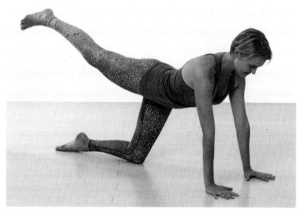

1. Start on all fours, with your hands under your shoulders and your knees under your hips. Walk both hands forward about 30cm (12in), to come to a kneeling Plank position.

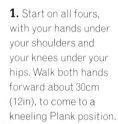

The exact distance will depend on your proportions, so aim to create a straight line from your knees through your hips to your shoulders. Roll your shoulders back, so that you broaden across your collar bones. This is an important action that you will aim to maintain for the whole sequence. Keep your shoulders nicely set by drawing your shoulder blades together slightly, as if magnetized. Lift your navel toward your spine. At the same time, create a sense of drawing your hip bones toward each other, across the front of the abdomen. Lift your right leg in the air behind you. Resist the urge to drop the abdomen toward the floor or to curve more into the lower back.

build up	**move forward**	**balance out**
Tiger Flow (page 32)	Crow to Plank Jump-Backs (page 148)	Yin Shoulder Stretches (page 322)

2. Check that the inner creases of both elbows are facing forward, then bend your elbows so that they brush past the sides of your waist. Keep your elbows snug into the side of your body, not splayed wide. Take your torso forward as you lower down, so that your fingertips will be level with your armpits. Think about going forward, rather than down to the ground. How much you lower is up to you. It's fine to drop just a little in the beginning. At your deepest you will create right-angles at the wrists and elbows. Straighten your arms to complete your push-up. Ensure your abdomen doesn't sag as you lift up. Check that your shoulders haven't rolled in, either. If you start to roll your shoulders in, then you have reached fatigue point and that means your body has had enough of this practice – work on it another day instead, and you will build up strength for deeper drops and more repetitions. Repeat five to ten more push-ups, paying attention to your form. Rest, and then complete a second set with your left leg lifted.

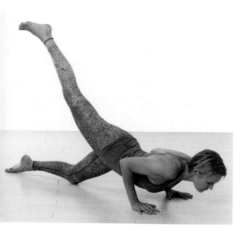

3. Once you have the strength to maintain good alignment, you can practise your yoga tricep push-ups with both knees off the floor and toes tucked under. If you have the strength, hold the low hover, just off the floor, in the full Crocodile pose.

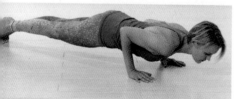

unwind
Basic Shoulder-Stand
(page 258)

take care
Rolling your shoulders in, or sagging at the belly, means it's time to rest. Seek advice if you have shoulder, elbow, wrist or neck pain.

classic crow

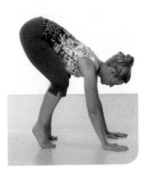

To freely balance in Crow Pose feels strong and empowering. Follow the alignment instructions carefully and your crow will soon fly.

1. From standing, fold forward and place your hands on the floor, shoulder width apart. Come onto tiptoes and walk your feet closer as you bend your knees, preparing to wrap them around your upper arms. You can tuck your knees up towards the armpits, or you may prefer to place them closer to your elbows. To prepare to bear more weight, reach your thumbs towards each other and spread your fingers wide. To protect your wrists, press into the floor with the pads of the fingers and thumbs.

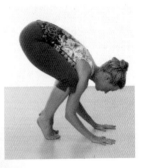
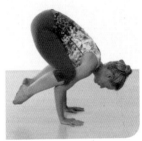

2. Notice how at this point your elbows are behind your wrists. The key to achieving Crow Pose is to bring your weight forward enough so the elbows stack above the wrists. This means being confident in your arm strength and ability to bend the elbows while bringing your shoulders forward and down. It is this action which will allow the feet to lift. Rather than trying to "hop" the feet up, just focus on bending the elbows to around 90 degrees while you move them forward above the wrists. Your head will drop a little towards the ground. As a by-product of all this, your feet will float effortlessly up in the air and you will have achieved Crow Pose. Stay for five to ten breaths.

STRONG NECK, STRETCHY SHOULDERS

build up
Open Squat Twist (page 178)

move forward
Crow to Plank Jump-Backs
(page 148)

balance out
Spine-Mobilizing Lunge
(page 42)

baby crow

I think this cute little version of the Crow Pose is ingenious. Not only does it save the wrists, but as it requires flexibility in the hips, it can be a nice option for anyone who is still building up to the full Crow balance.

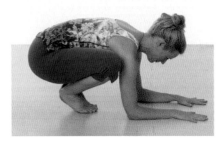 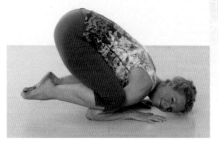

1. Take a low squat with the knees wide apart and the toes turned out. Fold at the hips, to lean the torso well forward. Move your ribcage as far forward between the thighs and as low down as possible. From this deep squat, walk your palms forward to allow you to bring your elbows to the floor, forearms parallel. Press the inner wrists and thumb knuckles down to the floor so they don't lift.

2. Now lift your hips higher as you rise up onto tiptoes to wrap your knees around the upper arms. Take your knees as high up as possible, pressing them to your outer arms. Draw up from the belly to create a strong centre. As you bend more at the elbows, tip your torso forward and lift your toes in the air to come into your forearm balance. It will feel a bit like nose-diving, so turn your head to the side. Hold for five to ten breaths. When we achieve a challenging pose, the mind can let go and the exit may be less dignified than the entry. Come out with mindfulness, reversing your moves to return to the low squat.

unwind
Classic Downward-Facing Dog Pose (page 58)

take care
Discontinue the pose and seek advice if it aggravates any existing neck, shoulder, elbow or wrist weakness or injury.

crow to plank jump-backs

Besides being a terrific workout for the arms and abdomen, Crow pose is great for the energy centre at the solar plexus. It builds mental focus, determination, strength and will power. Then success is yours for the taking.

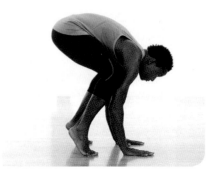

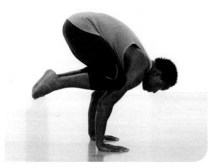

1. From standing, fold forward with bent knees to take your palms to the floor, shoulder-width apart and just under the shoulders. Turn your toes out and lift your heels to come onto tiptoes. Lift your hips and widen your knees apart, to wrap them around your upper-arm bones. There is a natural resting point for various body types – you might have your knees lower down, close to your elbows, or right up near your armpits.

2. Often the best way to lift your feet is to not think about them. As you bend your elbows, move your torso forward. This will ease your elbows forward and keep them sitting exactly above the wrist joints. At the same time, lower your shoulders toward elbow height. As you do this, your feet will float up into the air – there's no need to do any work to lift the toes. To help you balance, press your fingertips into the floor so that your forearm muscles activate. Experience your hands like a crow's feet "clawing" the earth. Balance here for several breaths.

build up	**move forward**	**balance out**
Crocodile Build-Up (page 144); Baby Crow (page 147)	Tripod to One-Legged Crow Pose (page 278)	Yin Shoulder Stretches (page 322)

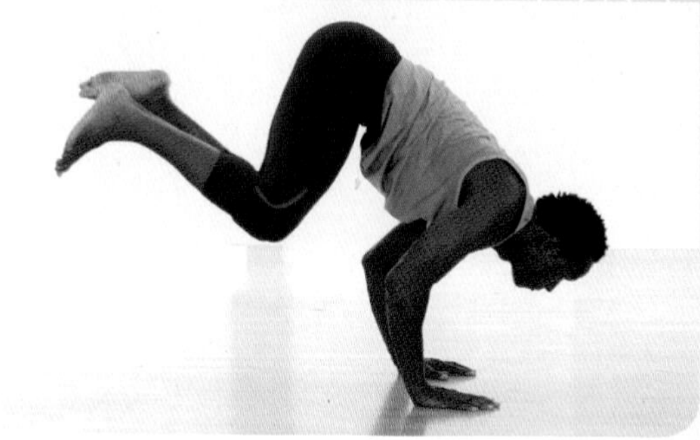

3. Now prepare for the jump-back. First, look forward rather than down. Squeeze your knees together to build the tension you will need initially, to propel yourself back. Prepare to shift your chest forward in the air, so that you will stay balanced over your hands for as long as possible. Now get ready to use your abdominal muscles to lift your hips up as you shoot your legs back. Be as symmetrical as possible with your legs as they perform this movement. Initially, this might be an explosive movement, but with practice and as your confidence builds, you will be able to slow it down, to "float" the legs gracefully back to a light landing.

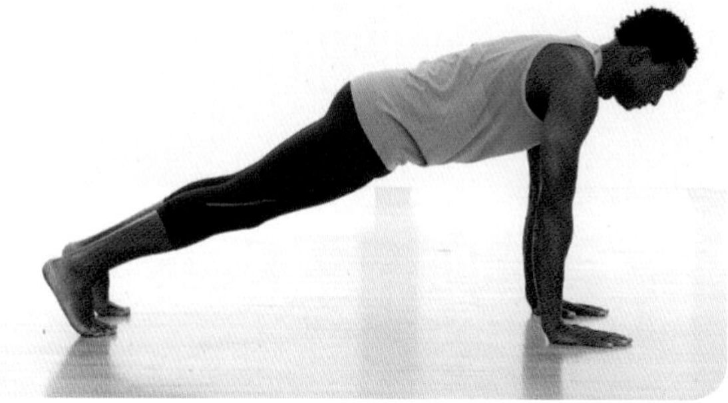

4. You are now in the Plank position. Take your awareness to the vertebrae between your shoulder blades and lift this area up to eradicate any gully between the shoulder blades. When you do this, it may feel as if it narrows the upper chest. To balance out this action, broaden across your collar bones and roll your shoulders back slightly. Hold the Plank position for five to ten breaths.

unwind

Corkscrew Twist (page 172)

take care

Discontinue the pose and seek advice if this aggravates any existing neck, shoulder, elbow or wrist weakness or injury.

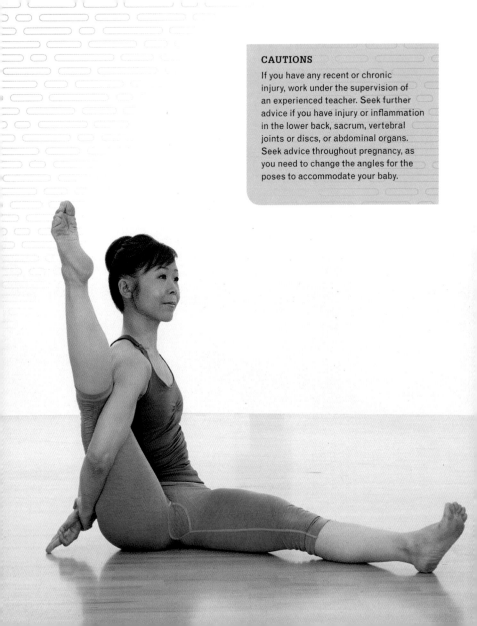

7

FLEXIBLE FORWARD FOLDS

Forward-folding postures feature heavily in yoga. They stretch out your whole back body – thighs, calves and back. They can help decompress the spine and relieve back pain and tension. They draw the awareness inward and can feel wonderful both during and afterward. And yes, life can feel better with looser hamstrings. It feels good to move with grace and pick up dropped items with ease.

But remember, even if your hamstrings don't lengthen as quickly as you wish, that yoga is actually a state of mind. If ever you catch yourself getting grumpy at your stubbornly short hamstrings, while forcing your nose to your knees, or comparing your flexibility to that of others, the best thing you can do is practise detachment and self-acceptance.

Keep in mind that it's not about measuring how *far* you go in a forward fold, but more about how *deeply* you can release for the duration. With floor-based postures, balance isn't generally an issue, so you have the opportunity to surrender to gravity rather than work against it. Don't invite struggle into your life – there's probably enough of that already, and it will only make your body tighten up more. Don't force your body to go where it's not ready to.

As forward bends are generally calming postures, practise surrendering to the present moment. Settle into your breath, honour the temple of your body and let it unfold in its own time. Don't measure your hamstrings; measure your ability to release. Develop self-acceptance and practise being content with where you are: right here, right now. That's yoga. And that's a practice you can really enjoy.

deep forward bend at the wall

One of my all-time favourite forward bends, this glorious pose will cleverly help you understand the dynamics of all the other forward folds.

1. Stand with your feet about 40cm (15in) from the wall. Have your feet hip-width apart, with your toes pointing forward. Lean your buttocks to the wall. The next movement might feel funny, but it's worth doing to get the most out of this pose. Reach one hand back to each buttock and, one at a time, tilt to pull the buttock flesh up and out to the side. This will allow you to nestle your sitting bones into the wall. Bend your knees, too, so that you can create the deepest possible forward fold at the hips. Take your fingertips to the floor in front, shoulder-width apart. Still with knees bent, work on finding the length from your pubic bone to your throat. On each inhalation your ribcage will float up a bit, which will create a little space. Then as you exhale you'll have the opportunity to release into this space, by reaching the heart centre forward to increase your stretch.

build up	**move forward**	**balance out**
East–West Flow (page 48)	Dancer's Bow (page 124)	Dancing Bridge (page 202)

2. As you hold, breathe and warm into the pose, and straighten your legs by sliding your sitting bones up the wall. This will increase the pelvic tilt, as will the angle of your legs. Sometimes we round the back and shut the breathing down a little in forward bends, but with the hands in front, you have a great opportunity to minimize that. You can use yoga blocks to help your body open further: walk your hands further forward to allow a really pleasant long and "flat" feeling along the front of the torso. If you don't have props handy, you can take your hands to the seat of a chair placed in front of you. After ten or more breaths, bend the knees and inhale to come up. Stand quietly to feel the effects of this pose.

unwind
Reclining Eagle Twist (page 226)

take care
Seek advice first from a professional in cases of slipped (herniated) disc or any inflammation of the back. Avoid inverted forward folds if you have a severe heart condition, high blood pressure, glaucoma, a detached retina, inner-ear discharge or a severe sinus infection.

kinky cobbler's pose

The special foot position of this pose adds a whole new element to this classic hip-opening forward bend. It turns it into a lovely stretch for those tight gluteal muscles, one side at a time.

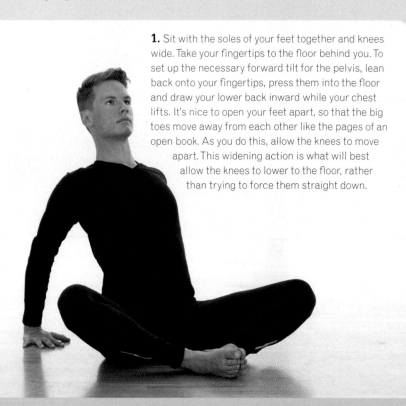

1. Sit with the soles of your feet together and knees wide. Take your fingertips to the floor behind you. To set up the necessary forward tilt for the pelvis, lean back onto your fingertips, press them into the floor and draw your lower back inward while your chest lifts. It's nice to open your feet apart, so that the big toes move away from each other like the pages of an open book. As you do this, allow the knees to move apart. This widening action is what will best allow the knees to lower to the floor, rather than trying to force them straight down.

build up
Head-Beyond-the-Knee Pose
(page 160)

move forward
Hip-Opening Heron Pose
(page 164)

balance out
Reclining Eagle Twist
(page 226)

FLEXIBLE FORWARD FOLDS

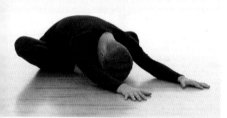

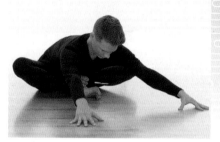

2. Now deepen the posture by rotating the pelvis forward even more. It's nice to maintain the thigh bones where they are, so think about the hip sockets moving forward around the head of the bones. If you can maintain the inward curve of the lower back, you can bring your fingertips to the floor in front and walk them away as you deepen the forward fold. If you find that your pelvis tilts backward as you let go of the floor behind you, you aren't yet ready for hands in front. Stay where you are for five to ten breaths.

3. Now add the release for the right buttock. Sit up and line up your right heel with your left toes. Starting with the hands behind once again, follow the same steps, moving into your deepest forward tilt. If you can, take your hands forward and walk them out front. Stay for five or ten long breaths, or for as long as you enjoy it. The come up and practise the other side.

unwind
Resting Cobbler's Poses
(page 284)

take care
If you suffer from sacroiliac pain, seek advice before doing this posture. Avoid it if you have a slipped disc.

tension-releasing forward fold

Nothing beats this pose for eradicating that build-up of tightness between the shoulder blades while working deeply into the hamstrings. When you come out of this pose, you will have had such a release of tension in the upper back that it will feel as if your whole world has changed – for the better, of course.

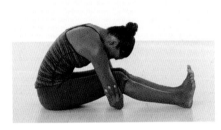 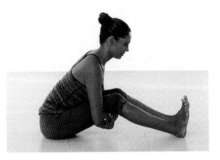

1. Sit with your knees bent up in front of you. Slide your forearms under your thighs and catch hold of each elbow. Now bring your spine into a well-rounded position. With your elbows held firmly, draw your ribs as far away from the fronts of your thighs as possible. Contract the abdominals into the lower back. Let your armpits move toward your elbows while you allow your shoulder blades to cleave away from each other. To assist with this rounding movement, tuck your tailbone under and draw your chin into your throat. Stay for several long breaths.

2. Now reverse the work. Lift your head and chest up as you flatten your back. Take your pelvis out of its backward tilt and into a forward tilt. Move your ribs forward and, as you lengthen the space between your front hip bones and your lowest ribs, your back will flatten. Now, with that flat-back feeling, exhale and close the gap by "laying" your belly and chest onto your thighs. Next, slide your feet forward slowly, until you feel your belly and chest wanting to separate from your thighs. Stop here and take five breaths.

build up
Easy Sun Salute (page 72)

move forward
Deep Forward Bend at the Wall
(page 152)

balance out
Half-Frog, Half-Locust
(page 236)

FLEXIBLE FORWARD FOLDS

3. Keeping your legs in their new further-away position, round your spine again while you create the most air space possible between your legs and your torso. "Give" your shoulders to your elbows while you separate your shoulder blades. Keep your chin in and your pelvis tucked under. Breathe! If you are very flexible, remove your forearms from under your legs to allow them to straighten completely, and clasp your heels.

Then reverse the pelvic tilt again and squash the air out from between your legs and torso by lengthening your torso from the pubic bone to the throat, flattening your back as much as possible. Keeping your abdomen and thighs together, slide your feet away some more. Repeat these two steps again. Come up, feel the difference and smile.

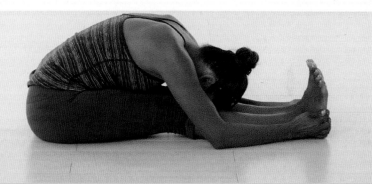

unwind
Banana Pose (page 194)

take care
Avoid this pose if you have had a slipped (herniated) disc.

heavenly happy-baby pose

This development on a classic Reclining Hand to Toe Pose will really take your hamstrings to new levels of flexibility, due to the clever use of pressing against a healthy resistance.

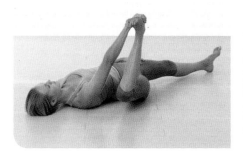

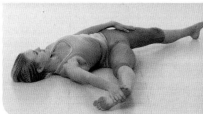

FLEXIBLE FORWARD FOLDS

1. Lie on your back with your knees bent up and your feet on the floor. Lift your right foot up and bring your knee in toward the right armpit. Clasp your inner heel with your right hand and press down, so that your thigh slides down past the side of your torso and your knee moves toward the floor. If that's not manageable, grab your ankle or shin, or loop a soft belt around your instep and hold that. If it feels comfortable, slide your left foot away, to add in a stretch for your left hip and thigh. Place your left palm on the top of that left thigh, to encourage it to ease down to the floor. Otherwise, keep your left knee bent up as you continue to step 2.

2. Now it's time to play with the resistance, which will bring a whole new quality to your stretch. Attempt to straighten your right knee while you continue to place pressure on your right heel. Try to bend your right elbow and, as you resist by pressing away with the leg, allow the leg to "win". Straighten the leg as much as you comfortably can, but maintain the resistance with your arm. This should feel like a deep but healthy stretch. After about ten breaths, come out and repeat this sequence on the second side.

build up	**move forward**	**balance out**
Hip-Releasing Wide Child Pose (page 216)	Half-Lotus Balance (page 166)	Three-up Bridge Pose (page 246)

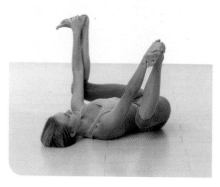

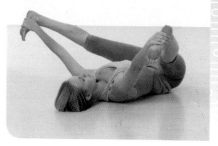

3. To come into the full Happy Baby, take both legs up, holding the heels. Tilt to one side, and then move back and forth, to rock your baby. This will encourage the hip-opening. Then settle into symmetry and enjoy your breathing. If your knees are close to the floor, add a degree of difficulty by bringing your pelvis into a forward tilt, as if to aim your tailbone closer to the floor and as if to pull your lower back away from the floor and into its natural curved shape. Hold and breathe while this stretch develops.

4. Now begin to straighten your legs as they move wide apart into a V-shape. Once again, resist with your arms, trying to bend your elbows, yet allow the legs to be victorious. If you can straighten your legs all the way, increase the challenge by changing your pelvic tilt, to lengthen your sitting bones down away from the heels and curve your lower back up slightly off the floor.

unwind
East–West Flow (page 48)

take care
If you ever feel a niggling pain or dull ache at either of your sitting bones after practising, seek further advice on working with forward bends. Work with an experienced teacher if you have had a disc injury.

head-beyond-the-knee pose

It's really worth taking time in the initial twisted stage of this pose, as it will set you up for a beautiful alignment in the final step.

1. Sit on the floor with your legs outstretched. Slide your right foot in and bring your knee out to the side. Place your toes roughly level with your left knee: take your foot slightly away from your inner leg, so that each heel is in front of its respective hip bone and both hips are fairly square-on to the front. Flex your ankle so that the "blade" of the foot – the little-toe edge – is in contact with the floor. If your hips are more open, bring your heel in toward your groin. In this position, more of the top of the foot will touch the ground. This option will allow for a deep release in the right side of the lower back.

After choosing your leg option, take your left hand behind you, and bring your right hand to the outer left thigh or knee. Inhale and float your spine tall as you twist to the left. The lower back will rotate better for you if it's in its natural convex shape, so be sure to press into the floor with your left hand to assist this curve. Squeeze your abdominal muscles toward the left, so that your pubic bone moves a little to the left. Stay in this upright twist for five to ten breaths.

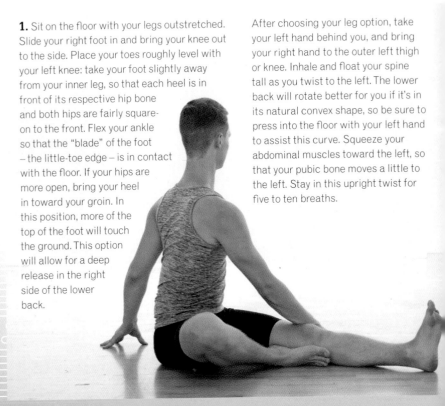

FLEXIBLE FORWARD FOLDS

build up
Standing Splits (page 122)

move forward
Half-Lotus Balance (page 166)

balance out
Flying Locust (page 38)

2. Maintaining the left-sided rotation of the torso, reach your right hand as far as possible down the left leg. Hold your foot, if you can. Bring your left hand to join the right. Due to the set-up twist, your shoulders can be level with each other. Breathe for five to ten long, slow breaths.

If you are flexible enough to reach, clasp your right wrist with your left hand and have the palm of the right hand facing away from you . Once you have a hold, press the ball of the foot away and enjoy the way this adds to the stretch in the shoulders. Repeat to practise side two.

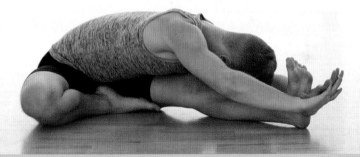

unwind
East–West Flow
(page 48)

take care
Take the first leg-positioning option at step 1 if you are prone to sacroiliac dysfunction or if your ankle ligaments are lax. Sit your hips on a folded blanket or cushion to assist the forward fold if you feel tight. Avoid forward folds if you have disc issues, and instead build up to them under the care of a physiotherapist.

seated rotated gate

This is a lovely sequence to relieve lower-back tightness, as each stage squeezes and stretches tensions out of the opposite side of the back. It also works into so many people's favourite tight places – the hips and hamstrings.

1. Sit with your left leg outstretched. Taking your right foot behind you, bend your right knee out to the side so that your thighs are perpendicular to each other. Ensure the top of your right foot is in contact with the floor. Your toes will point toward your right buttock. Take your left hand to your right outer knee and your right fingertips to the floor behind your back. Draw yourself up to create a dignified elegance. Then you will be ready to twist to the right. Involve your abdominal muscles in this twist, so that they squeeze around to the right. In addition, your arms will act as levers to spiral you round. Consciously activate the muscles of the mid- and upper back to draw you further round another notch or two. Stay for five to ten breaths.

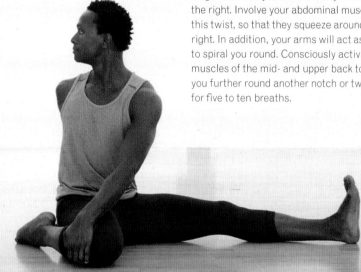

build up
Pyramid Prayer (page 140)

move forward
Hip-Opening Heron Pose
(page 164)

balance out
Cobbler's Bridge (page 192)

2. Now change the direction of your twist by taking both hands to the floor, one on either side of your left leg. Revolve your lower abdominals as far to the left as possible. Walk your hands away a little, so that the forward stretch is not too intense. Find your beautiful alignment before you deepen the intensity: taking an inhalation, lift your front ribs up and away from your hips. This will create space in your body and help flatten your back. Then, as you exhale, move your belly button forward and down the left thigh, to close the space between your midriff and your leg. Maintaining a sense of length from your pubic bone to your throat, walk your hands away, grasping the foot, if possible. Hold for five to ten breaths.

3. Come on up and return to the upright right-sided twist. Stay for several long breaths, then unravel and repeat the long forward fold over your left leg. Enjoy the sense of your body opening, with this chance to revisit and deepen these two postures. Then practice side two.

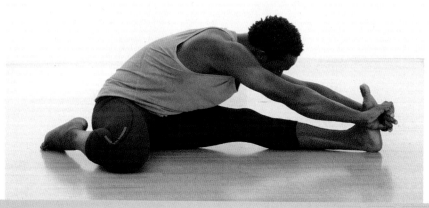

unwind
Cow-Pose Spirals (page 222)

take care
Sit your hips on a folded blanket or cushion to assist the forward fold, if you feel tight. Avoid forward folds if you have disc issues, and instead build up to them under the care of a physiotherapist.

hip-opening heron pose

☆
☆
☆

This deep forward fold requires hamstring flexibility and strength. It's a clever one, as the muscle activation required in the front of the thigh of your raised leg assists the release in the back of that thigh to help it lengthen, allowing you to achieve the pose.

1. Warm up your hip first by cradling your right lower leg; you can simply slip your bent elbows under your calf as you slowly rock it from side to side, like a baby, or you can cup the knee and foot in your hands and press them toward each other. Don't collapse into your lower back – pull the lower back into its natural curve and feel how your chest lifts as you sit tall. As your hip releases, close the gap between your shin and chest. If you can, lift your foot higher.

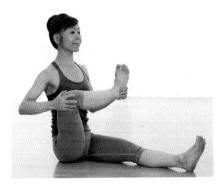

2. Ease your right knee back behind your right armpit. Hunch over forward a little and position your right upper arm under your right thigh, to help press the knee back another little bit and find that hip-opening action even more. Then undo any slouching, to sit as tall as possible again. Place your right palm on the floor beside, or if possible behind, your buttock. Take your left hand to your right foot.

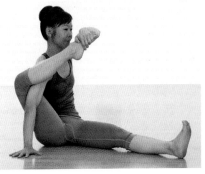

build up	**move forward**	**balance out**
Bound Side-Angle Stretch (page 104)	Yin Dragon Lunge (page 320)	Twisted Pigeon (page 182)

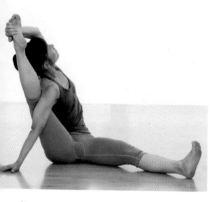 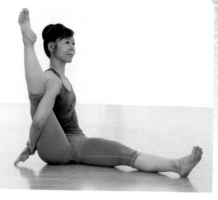

3. You are now ready to straighten your right leg by pressing your right foot into your left hand to lift it up into the air. With the right upper arm jammed into the back of the leg (to maintain the hip-opening position), this means that you have to squeeze on the muscles of your right front thigh to get the leg as straight as possible. Press the floor away with your right hand, as you turn your torso and head upward, to gaze up. If you feel good here, go for the arm lock in step 4.

4. Release your right hand from the floor and, rotating from the shoulder, turn your palm outward. Your elbow will bend and lift up. Slide the back of your hand under your right thigh and place it against your sacrum. Similarly, release your left hand and rotate the palm out, thumb down. The elbow will bend up and allow your left hand to slide down to the lower back. Grasp your left wrist with your right hand. Straighten your elbows as much as possible, lift your chest and straighten your right knee. After several breaths, release and practise side two.

unwind
Reclining Eagle Twist
(page 226)

take care
Avoid forward folds if you have disc issues, and instead build up to them under the care of a physiotherapist.

half-lotus balance

☆
☆
☆

It's fun to bring the challenge of balance and core-strengthening to this hip-opening forward bend.

1. To prepare your hip for the Half-Lotus, sit on the floor and take your right leg up to cradle the baby, like step 1 of the Hip-Opening Heron Pose on page 164. Once you feel warmed up, bend your right knee out to the side, to place your right ankle as high up your left thigh as possible. Snuggle your right heel into the left groin. This is a Half-Lotus position. Don't hold this pose if there is any discomfort in your knee; instead, come out and move on to the "Happy Hips" section (see pages 214–27) to develop the flexibility in your hips. If your knee feels fine, then stay here, allowing the knee to drop lower as the right hip releases. To help prepare for the balancing forward fold, take a Half-Lotus Forward Fold by bending over the left leg while it's grounded. Again, check that there is no discomfort in the bent knee while you hold for a full minute, breathing slowly and evenly.

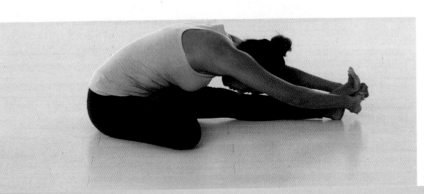

build up
Head-Beyond-the-Knee Pose
(page 160)

move forward
Seated Yogic Roll-Downs
(page 204)

balance out
Yoga Swimming Bow (page 240)

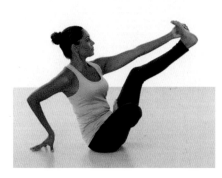

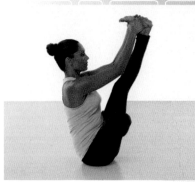

2. Sitting upright, slide your left foot in as you bend the left knee up and slightly out to the left. Reach forward to catch your left foot with both hands. Grasp your calf or ankle, if you can't reach the foot.

3. Straighten your left leg up into the air, as you bring that knee more to the centre. Close the gap between your torso and your legs while you balance, and take the stretch as deep as feels great. Hold for five to ten breaths.

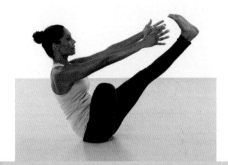

4. Now let go of your leg and extend your arms out to horizontal. Lean back, curving your spine into a C-shape, and work your abdominal muscles. To increase the strengthening effect, lower your legs away to create more of a boat shape. Hold for six breaths or longer, until you feel your abdominals fatiguing with the effort.

HALF-LOTUS BALANCE

unwind
Reclining Eagle Twist
(page 226)

take care
Warm up your hips before attempting this pose, and come out if there is any knee pain. If you have a history of a slipped disc, seek advice before trying it.

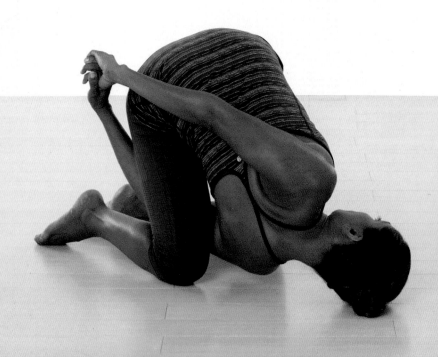

8

JUICY TWISTS

Twists may appear less glamorous or exciting than some other yoga poses, but they offer enormous health benefits. Yogis understand that having a flexible spine feels a bit like tapping into the fountain of youth. As twists increase your spinal range of motion, they not only keep you looking young, but *feeling* young, too. Some of the aims in yoga, when working with the spine, are to strengthen and stabilize it, mobilize it, allow it to relax and lengthen, and to create differentiation.

A twist can tick all these boxes. It can work wonders for back pain and it also aids the digestive process. Like the yoga side-stretches, twists are great counterposes after forward bends and backbends. And they are excellent preparatory poses, too, making any subsequent pose more accessible.

Twists can feel like an amazing tonic for your nervous system. They bring you back into balance and help neutralize the fluctuations of the mind. Twists work whether you are feeling stressed-and-wired or stressed-and-tired. If you are feeling heavy, fatigued or mentally sluggish, twists give you a lift, helping you feel refreshed, buoyant and energized. Try a therapeutic twist next time you have a mid-afternoon slump. However, if you are feeling scattered, fragmented and can't focus, twists will ground you and bring you "home", much closer to the calm and peaceful self that always resides within.

☆ three-step reclining twist

What's great about reclining twists is that the paraspinal muscles can relax. Because, when you are lying down, your vertebral column doesn't have to work against gravity, it feels easier to lengthen it. After using the three stages here, you will mobilize better, as you'll be twisting into different areas of the spine.

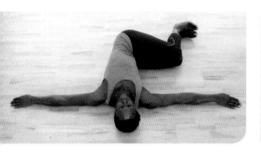 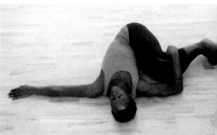

1. Lie on your back with your knees bent up, and your feet on the floor. Take your arms out wide, with your hands at shoulder level. Your palms can be up or down, whichever you prefer. To keep your spine more even in the twist, lift your hips and move them 5cm (2in) to the left side.

2. Now bend your knees into your chest. Wrap your right arm around both shins and use it to guide your legs all the way to the right, so that the thighs stay as close as possible to your torso. Once on the floor, ease your right arm out from under your legs and drape it over the top leg. Press your left shoulder toward the earth, and slide it and your left hand further to the left to increase the stretch. Find the position that feels nicest for your neck: looking right, up or left. Allow all the work to stop, let everything go and feel deliciously heavy. Stay for ten or 15 breaths.

build up
Shoulder Sweeps (page 34)

move forward
Revolved Bound Lunge
(page 92)

balance out
Seated Yogic Roll-Downs
(page 204)

3. Now move the emphasis of the twist further down the spine. Take your thighs away from the torso and create right-angles at the hips and the knees. Your feet will be in a line straight down from your knees. Your knees will fall in the straight line

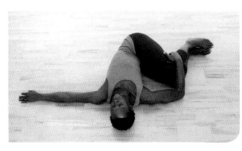

extending out from the hips. Allow your top knee to sit a little behind your lower knee. If your lower back is strong and you would like to develop the twist, press your top knee forward so that both knees stack, as you earth your left shoulder down. Check your head position to make sure your neck is happy in this pose and breathe for eight to 15 rounds.

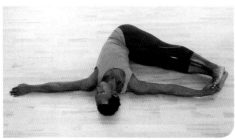

4. Now move to a more active twist. Bend the knees in close and cup your right palm over both sets of toes. If this isn't manageable, grasp a soft belt looped around the balls of the feet. Straighten your legs as much as possible while aiming the feet toward shoulder level. Stack your top heel over the bottom heel. Use that as an anchor point and set up a radiation in the direction of your left hand. Squeeze your abdominals to the left to allow your left shoulder to ground down. Ease your left shoulder toward your left hand. Stay for eight or more breaths. Come out and, starting from the centre, work through the second side.

THREE-STEP RECLINING TWIST

unwind
Gate Pose Flow (page 188)

take care
Seek advice for all twists and forward bends if you are at risk of disc herniation, and don't practise this if you have had active symptoms recently. Work with a strong core if you have pelvic imbalance. Avoid strong twists with some inflammatory digestive conditions.

☆ corkscrew twist

This cute little pose is a twist – with a twist. As your core muscles are not being used to hold you upright, it means that you can relax really nicely for the first part. The second part offers you a lovely squeezy massage-feeling around the abdominal organs, with a little increased pressure.

1. Lie on your back with your knees bent into your chest. Rest your right arm on your shins and hug your knees in close. Use your abdominal muscles to help draw the thighs in. Then guide your legs to the right so that they rest on the floor, with your knees as close to your armpit as possible. Place your right arm across your knees, to remind the hip and thigh muscles to soften. Then find the most luxurious position for your left arm. You can bend the elbow and place your palm on your ribs, but most people like to have their back arm out to the side, palm up. To give the side of your torso a little more release, slide your arm higher up so that it's closer to your ear. Now seek out the nicest way to position your head and neck. First close your eyes, then very slowly move your head from looking to the right over toward the left. Somewhere along the route there will be a happy 'Ahhh' feeling, signalling where your neck likes to be. It's often different on each side.

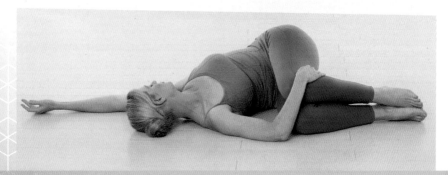

build up
Spine-Mobilizing Lunge
(page 42)

move forward
Twisted Pigeon (page 182)

balance out
Dancing Bridge (page 202)

JUICY TWISTS

172

2. Once you are comfortable, settle in and stay there for a minute or so. Turn your focus to any areas of the body that are tight and encourage them to release. Consider the usual suspects – back, shoulders, neck – but also roam freely. Is there any tension holding in the soles of the feet? How are the buttocks? What about your jaw? Bringing awareness to tight or tender areas starts the path of healing and softening.

To move into a feeling of actively spiralling, lift your feet up, angling your shins to point both knees downward. This will activate the oblique muscles of your core. Recommit your left shoulder to the floor. This will also impact on your breathing – it might feel shorter or less smooth. Bring mindfulness to your breath so that it can round out more. Stay for five to eight breaths. Then practise side two.

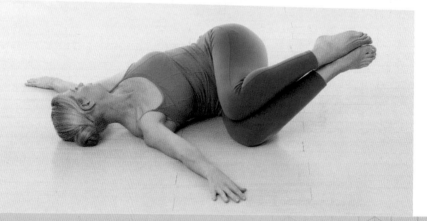

unwind
Backbend Ripple (page 290)

take care
Seek advice for all twists and forward bends if you are at risk of disc herniation. Work with a strong core if you have pelvic imbalance.

revolved happy pose

The four-step process detailed here can be used in every twist you will ever attempt, and it will really take your twisting to a whole new level. You always want to elongate the spine first, and you generally want to twist from your base up. Go forth and conquer the marvellous world of twists.

1. Sit in an easy cross-legged pose. If you feel stiff, sit on a cushion to lift your hips in relation to your knees. If cross-legged doesn't work for you, try kneeling with your knees apart or together. Cup your right knee with your left hand and find a good spot on the floor, somewhere out from your tailbone, to place your right palm or fingertips. The first step of your twist is to think about your lower abdomen. Elongate as you take a full inhalation, then on an exhale switch on your abdominal muscles and direct them firmly to the right. Notice how far you move during this first stage of your rotation. It will be a combination of strength in the torso muscles and the work of both arms.

2. Inhale and draw yourself tall once again. As you exhale, squeeze the upper abdomen around to the right to rotate further. Keep your belly muscles on, so that they draw inward to your centre.

3. Your abdomen will feel tight and strong, so you will feel your next inhalation more in the chest. As you breathe in, allow the chest to lift, and then exhale and move it as much as possible into your twist.

4. Finally, think of your shoulders. Inhale and lengthen from tailbone to crown, then exhale and move both shoulders further into the twist. On an exhalation, come out of the twist – as you do so, you may feel a release of pressure, like opening a bottle of sparkling water. Enjoy these bubbles of release while you sit symmetrically. Then work with the second side, again working from bottom to top. Try this four-step bottom-to-top process in other twists, such as the Cow-Pose Spirals, as shown on page 222.

JUICY TWISTS

build up	**move forward**	**balance out**	**unwind**
Spine Mobilizer (page 50)	Intense Reclining Side-Stretch (page 196)	Seated Yogic Roll-Downs (page 204)	Tiger Flow (page 32)

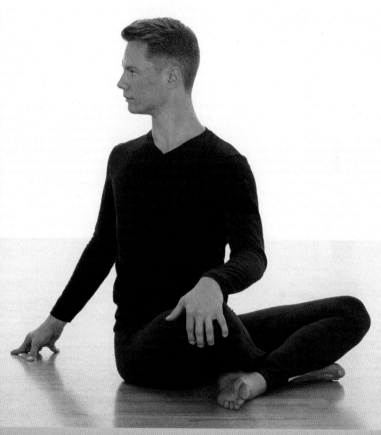

take care

Seek advice for all twists if you are at risk of disc herniation. If you have sacroiliac dysfunction, don't attempt to keep your hips square to the front. Instead, as you twist to the right, slide your left buttock forward a little and allow your right hip to move back in relation to the left hip. Don't over-tighten the abdominal muscles in pregnancy. Avoid strong twists with some inflammatory digestive conditions.

sage pose with neck releases

These ingenious neck releases are easily incorporated into most twists, and people fall in love with the sensations they offer. They are strong, though, so remember that less is more when it comes to stretching the neck and go gently until you become acquainted with how your neck responds.

1. For Sage Pose, first sit and bring both feet around to the left. Have the toes of your left foot pointing straight back, and place your right foot over the instep of the left. You will feel a natural tipping to the right, so do your best to snuggle your left buttock down toward the floor. If you feel too lopsided, level the hips more by lifting your seat. To level out, sit on a folded blanket or a yoga block. Rotating to your right side, take your left hand to the right knee and position your right fingertips on the floor behind you. Use your arms as levers to help you come into a deep and satisfying twist.

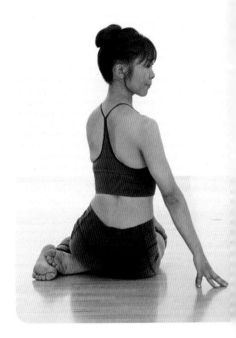

build up	**move forward**	**balance out**	**unwind**
Magical Shoulder and Neck Release (page 136)	Threaded Needle (page 180)	Three-Up Bridge Pose (page 246)	Kinky Cobbler's Pose (page 154)

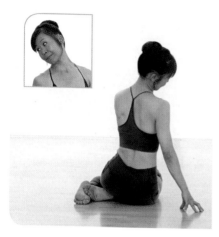

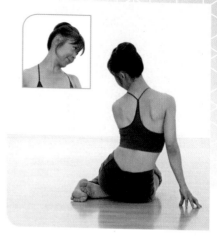

2. Once you are settled in your twist, set up your first neck stretch. Starting from a neutral head position, where your jawline is parallel to the floor, rotate your head to the right so that you are looking behind you. Ensure it feels comfortable. Now, tilt your head by dropping your right earlobe down to your right shoulder. Bring your chin closer to your throat. Now squeeze on the muscles by your armpits, to lower your left shoulder. Experience a fairly strong diagonal line of stretch along the left side of your neck. If you wish, create a tiny nodding action. Stay for three to five long breaths.

3. Stay in the twist, but return your head and neck to a neutral position. Keeping a sense of elongation in the neck, swivel your head to the left, so that you are looking over your left shoulder. First tilt the face downward a small amount, tucking the chin in. Then drop your left ear down. Accentuate the stretch along the neck and back shoulder by lowering the right shoulder. Hold for five breaths, then release the head to neutral. Come out of the twist and stretch your legs out in front of you. Take a moment to check in with how your neck feels. Then swing your legs to the right, ready to practise the second side.

take care

If you have a history of neck injury or tightness, use only half the effort during your first experiences of this practice, and build up the intensity of effort and length of stay over time.

Avoid strong twists with some inflammatory digestive conditions. Seek advice if you have sacroiliac dysfunction.

open squat twist

In this lovely twist you can use your reaching arm to encourage a delightful sense of lengthening in the spine. For the more adept, the looping action really gives a great squeezy massage to tight muscles, so it feels amazing.

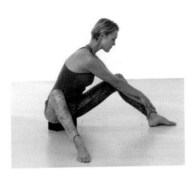

1. A great adjunct to this pose is to raise your seat by sitting on a foam brick or a blanket folded four times. Sit on your support, or on the floor, and bend your knees up in front. Place your feet a little wider than your shoulders and turn your toes out. This will allow your knees to ease away from each other, so that you get an inner-thigh stretch as well. Hold your left shin, ankle or, if possible, foot with your left hand. Tap your right hand to your left, then reach your right hand out and up in a wide arc.

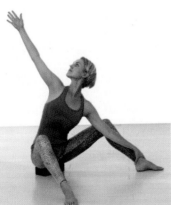

2. Make sure your abdominal section is involved in this twist. Your core muscles will switch on, to help the rotation from your solar plexus. Combined with the elevating reach of your right arm, you may feel a diagonal pull as the upper right part of your abdomen moves away from your lower left side. Anchor yourself by pressing your left arm to your left leg. Then come alive through your centre, as you continue to radiate your right arm up and away. Hold for five to ten breaths, then rest.

build up
Side-Angle Pose (page 186)

move forward
Twisted Pigeon (page 182)

balance out
Seated Yogic Roll-Downs (page 204)

JUICY TWISTS

3. To come into the loop, slide your left armpit down to your left inner thigh, just before the knee. It will feel as if this shortens the left side of the torso, but it's all part of the contract-and-release benefits of a twist: some parts of you will condense, others will expand. Once your left shoulder is as low as it can go, rotate from your shoulder in order to slide your left forearm under your left thigh, then bring the back of your hand across until it rests on your sacrum.

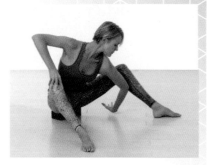

4. With your lower arm locked in place, reach your upper arm up and away, as in step 1. Rotating from the shoulder, turn your right thumb forward and down. As you bend your elbow up, bring

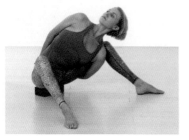 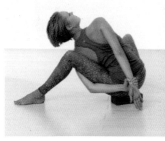

your right hand low, to slide the back of it across your lower back. Curl your fingers to lock the hands together or, if you can, grasp your right wrist with your left hand. If you can't reach, complete the loop between both hands by holding a soft belt.

5. To add that extra bit to your twist, and to accentuate the shoulder and hip stretches, send a current of energy through both elbows to straighten them. As you do this, move your hands away from your body, so that eventually your hands don't touch your body at all. Stay for five breaths. Then repeat on the second side.

OPEN SQUAT TWIST

---

unwind
Seated Rotated Gate
(page 162)

take care
Avoid twists if you are at risk of disc herniation. Avoid strong twists during pregnancy or with some inflammatory digestive conditions.

threaded needle

It's always satisfying when you can sneak a great shoulder release into any pose. The shoulder-stretching work during this bind really develops the twist beautifully. Enjoy!

1. Starting on your hands and knees, inhale and reach your right arm up in the air. As you exhale, sweep your right arm out wide and down, to slide your forearm under your left armpit. Your left elbow will bend on this downward movement, allowing you to snuggle your right shoulder to the floor. Repeat three to five times, inhaling as your right arm moves through a wide upward arc and exhaling each time you "thread the needle".

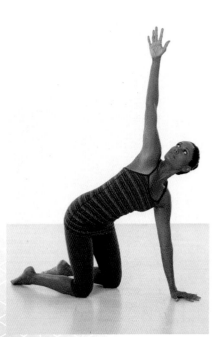

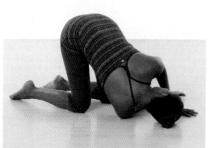

build up	**move forward**	**balance out**
Open Squat Twist (page 178)	Reclining Eagle Twist (page 226)	Dancing Bridge (page 202)

2. To move into the fully threaded needle, you will be bringing your right arm through your inner thighs. Set up this movement from your all-fours starting position by rolling your right shoulder forward, so that your elbow lifts up and your palm faces right. As you slide your forearm through the legs, the blade of the little-finger end of your hand will be closest to the floor. Bend your left elbow to allow your head and right shoulder to rest to the floor. Slide the back of your right hand as high up as possible, to rest against your right buttock. Now lift your left arm up into the air and, rotating through the shoulder, bend the elbow and turn your palm backward, thumb down. Slide the back of the hand across your lower back and lock the fingers of both hands. A common error is to loop the hands around the left buttock, so check that you have looped around the more challenging right hip. If possible, hold your left wrist with your right hand. Juice up this twist by straightening as much as possible through the elbows. Try not to touch your buttock with your hands, as your shoulders press away from the ears. After at least five breaths, come out. Kneel to sit symmetrically and feel the differences in your body. Repeat on the second side.

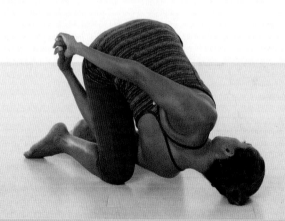

unwind
Prayer Sweeps (page 206)

take care
Avoid twists if you are at risk of disc herniation. Avoid strong twists during pregnancy or with some inflammatory digestive conditions.

twisted pigeon

This pose combines a terrific twist with a valuable stretch for the external hip rotator and gluteal muscles. As you twist in each direction, it offers different releases through the hips, abdomen and ribcage.

1. Kneel on all fours and bring your left shin forward between your hands. If you feel comfortable, position your left foot further forward, so that your shin is more perpendicular to your body. If you are less flexible, your left knee will point forward while your left foot will be closer to your right hip. Slide your right leg as far back and away as possible. If your left buttock doesn't touch the floor, place a yoga brick or folded blanket underneath it: you should feel able to lift both hands without any major shift occurring while your hips settle into this stretch. Press your palms to the floor and enjoy the way your spine curves into a long, upward-lifting sweep. Now take your twist to the right. With your left hand placed on your left knee or the ground nearby, reach your right hand to the back of your right leg. Lift tall each time you inhale, then revolve a little more each time you exhale. Imagine a pleasant squeeze through the right lower back and kidney area. Enhance that by sliding your right fingers further down the leg. Choose whether you prefer to allow your right hip bone to slide back, taking it with you into the twist, or whether you would like to increase the intensity by pressing it forward as if to square the hips. Hold for at least five breaths.

build up
Pigeon Pose with
Scientific Stretching
(page 224)

move forward
Pigeon Crescent Pose
(page 242)

balance out
Yin Happy Baby
(page 318)

unwind
Resting Cobbler's
Poses (page 284)

JUICY TWISTS

2. Return to face forward, ready to twist to the left. Relax your hips toward the floor. Position your right hand to the floor in front or, if you can, on your left knee. Reach around with your left hand and slide the back of the hand across your lower back. Rotate your palm down to hold your clothing, or cup it across your right hip. If your left foot is near that hip, it might even be possible for you to loop your thumb and first two fingers around your big toe. Hold for five breaths or more. Then release out of the pose, ready for side two.

take care

Avoid twists if you are at risk of disc herniation. If you experience knee pain, try using the support of a bolster or folded blankets under the front thigh, to lift the hip higher than your knee. Avoid strong twists with some inflammatory digestive conditions. Take it easy during pregnancy and don't over-tighten the abdominal muscles.

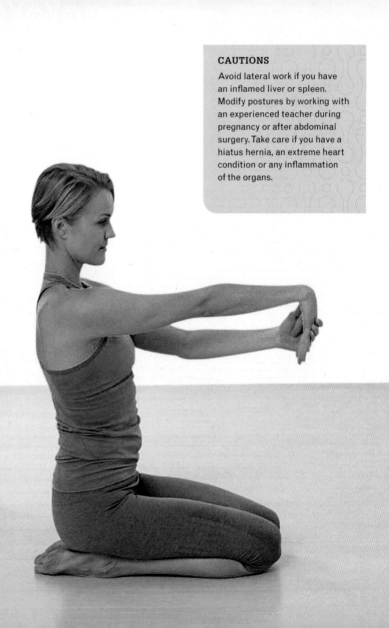

9

STRONG, STRETCHY SIDES

In some ways lateral stretches are the unsung heroes of yoga practice. We don't seem to really stretch our side-bodies much in our day-to-day lives, so to do so during yoga can feel amazing – like opening the door to a previously undiscovered room in a mansion. With yoga practice you will shine the light into this room. It may be a little musty, but use these postures to dust it off and you will find that your whole body runs a little better.

As a valuable part of our core unit, side-body strengtheners help our stability, power and balance. But you don't only want strength – you need the stretching, too. Lateral releases are invaluable for stretching out tight lower backs. They are great twist-enhancers, bring backbends along like magic, allow your breathing to blossom, make you feel taller and give you a more elegant posture.

You will find lots of other side-body stretches and strengtheners throughout this book. But read on for some favourite ways to work with this group of postures and enjoy discovering how they will be champions for your body.

☆ side-angle pose

The directional breathing featured here really helps hard and tense bodies to reset themselves, so you will feel open and soft again. And moving through the world with a softer and more open body feels so much better than navigating your way with excess tension and tightness.

1. Step your feet 1.2–1.5m (4–5ft) apart. You'll choose the wider range if you have longer or more flexible legs. Moving from the thigh, turn your right foot in by about 15 degrees. With your left toes pointing straight out to the left, bend your left knee so that it sits above your left ankle. To come into the first stage, reach your left elbow to your left knee and take your right arm up to vertical. Rotating from the shoulder joint, turn your right palm to the left and extend your arm to hover above your right ear.

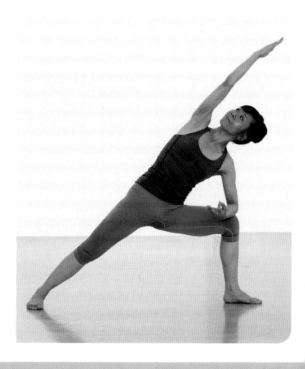

build up
Exultant Warrior Flow (page 98)

move forward
Bowing Side-Angle Pose
(page 100)

balance out
Head-Beyond-the-Knee Pose
(page 160)

STRONG, STRETCHY SIDES

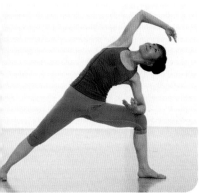

2. Now finesse the side-stretch. First, ease off the reach through the top arm. Bend your top elbow, and allow your right forearm and wrist to flop. Lift your right elbow straight up and also away from your right hip. Now, in a subtle shift of about 5cm (2in), slide your left hip toward the left and deepen the arc from left hip to left armpit, further increasing the length through the right side of the lower back. Finally, imagine that you are a fish, using its side-gills to breathe. Visualize your breath moving in and out of your right-side ribs, as if it were bypassing your nose.

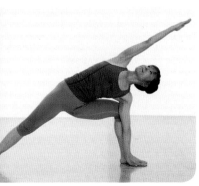

3. If you would like to go deeper, take the left palm to the floor. Choose whether to straighten your right arm to form the classic Side-Angle Pose or continue to work with the elbow to fingertips nicely floppy. Enjoy breathing in and out of your right "gills" for several more breaths. Each slow, deep intake of air will stretch the little muscles in between the ribs, as the ribcage expands. This will reset your breathing, so that you can breathe slower and deeper, which will help you feel more relaxed. It sets up a cycle of positive reinforcement: as you relax more, you breathe more slowly; then, as you breathe more slowly, you can relax more. Who would have thought that breathing like a fish could feel so nourishing? Then come back up, to work the second side.

unwind
Backbend Ripple (page 290)

take care
Ensure that your knee sits above or behind the ankle below, and don't let it move in front of the ankle.

☆ gate pose flow

This sequence uses the initial twisting action to free up the body, to improve the quality of the lateral stretch that follows. The supportive head-hold will allow the rest of the body to feel safe enough to work deeper into the stretch. The progressive lengthening action is a really nice one to know about because, once you understand the principles, it can be applied to just about any yoga pose for the rest of your life.

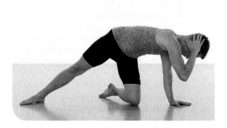 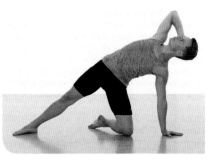

1. From kneeling, take your right leg out so that the right foot is level with your left knee. Have your toes reaching away to the right. Lift up all your toes, fan them apart, then place them on the floor, stretched out wide. Really move them away from each other, as if they were greedy for extra spce. Lean to the left as you place your left fist or palm on the floor, also in line with your left knee. Take your right hand behind your head to cup the base of your skull. Position your hold so that you can take as much load off the neck as possible.

2. Add a flowing twist to this side-stretch. Revolving from the lower abdomen, exhale and turn your torso toward the floor, while your top elbow moves forward. Inhale and spiral through the torso as your elbow moves to the sky. Continue exhaling to close, and inhaling to open, for several more rounds.

build up
Dragon Flow (page 46)

move forward
Intense Reclining Side-Stretch
(page 196)

balance out
Half-Frog, Half-Locust
(page 236)

STRONG, STRETCHY SIDES

3. Once you are facing forward again, release the head support and lengthen your right arm up and over to the left with your palm facing down.

4. Work systematically now, to "grow" a little. Press down through those widely spread right toes again, particularly through the big-toe knuckle and the whole ball of the foot. These will be your anchor points. Now start to progressively create a strong line of energy along the whole of the right side. Lift up from your right ankle toward your right knee. Then firm the quadriceps, so that the kneecap lifts toward your right hip. Lift and lengthen

your side-ribs up and away from your right hip. Then reach your armpit away from your waist. Firm your upper-arm muscles to the arm bone, and move your elbow away from your shoulder. Visualize little pockets of space being created in these joints. Next, move your wrist away from your elbow. Spread the skin on the palm of your hand as you fan your fingers away. Lengthen through each finger and your thumb, again sensing space being made in each of these little joints. Breathe, expand and enjoy, before working with the second side.

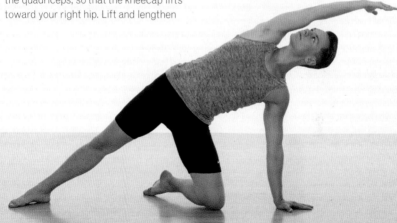

unwind
Resting Pigeon (page 294)

take care
Place a folded blanket under the knee for padding, if you need to.

inclined plane pose

This pose strengthens the muscles of the side-waist. Yoga aficionados can be a little weak in this area, as many yoga postures stretch out the sides more than strengthening them. So do yourself a favour and bring a little energy to these muscles. You will appreciate the benefits as you walk tall, as if you are gliding with grace.

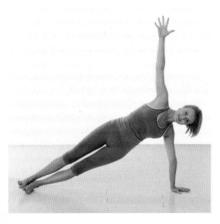

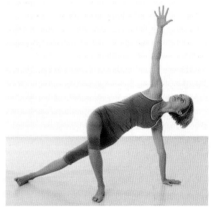

1. From the Plank position (see page 77, step 5), sway your heels to the left. Press through your left hand as you lift your right arm up to vertical. At the same time, lift your right hip to stack both hips in one line. Ensure that your weight-bearing shoulder draws down away from the ear. In yoga, we don't like to wear the shoulders as earrings.

2. You are aiming to rest your weight on the little-toe blade of your left foot, with your right foot lined up on top. A slightly easier option is to position the top foot in front of the bottom foot, heel to toe. If you don't yet have the strength for this, you can bend your top knee and place your right foot on the floor in front of your left knee, as shown.

build up	**move forward**	**balance out**
Seated Yogic Roll-Downs (page 204)	Core-Activating Plank Flow (page 212)	Seated Rotated Gate (page 162)

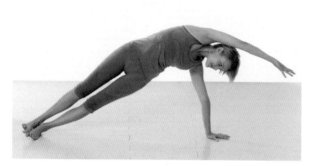
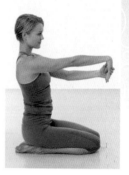

3. From your starting point as a flat line from feet through hips to shoulders, now create an arch. Work the muscles of your waist to lift your hips up and curve your shape. This will take some of the load off the shoulder and will work your oblique abdominals more. Do this on the exhalation and, as you inhale, return to your straight line. If you can manage it, reach your arm overhead to form part of the curve each time you exhale, then return it up to vertical on your inhalation. Continue contracting your waist away from the floor and slowly lifting to curve as you exhale, while lowering with control and mindfulness on your inhalations. Complete five rounds.

4. Then come down and sit back. Offer your wrists a counterpose by curling your fingers down as if to tickle your forearms. You are now ready to work side two.

unwind
Restorative Twist (page 292)

take care
Build up your wrist strength with Plank and Downward-Facing Dog practice.

cobbler's bridge

This hip-opening backbend, inspired by Japanese yoga therapy, strengthens the back, inner thigh, hamstring and buttock muscles. It is also a terrific route to developing your core muscles in a flowing, organic way.

1. Lie on your back with your arms just wide from the hips, palms down. Bring the soles of your feet together. Allow your knees to drop apart from each other. This is usually a yoga signal for the body to relax, so take a few long, slow breaths to enjoy this position before you begin your strength work.

2. To prepare to lift up, press the soles of the feet together actively. Squeeze your buttock muscles and, keeping your knees wide, lift your hips as high as possible off the floor. Roll your shoulders under to give more lift to the chest. Feel your back muscles working strongly to keep you in an arched shape.

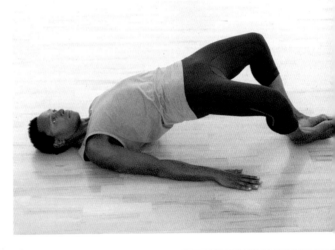

STRONG, STRETCHY SIDES

build up
Prayer Sweeps (page 206)

move forward
Plough-Pose Lifts (page 208)

balance out
Yin Happy Baby (page 318)

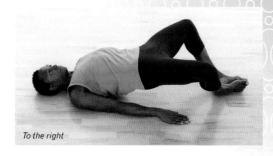

To the right

3. Take an inhalation and then, on each exhalation, shunt your hips from side to side. When you breathe in, return to the middle; when you breathe out, slide to the side. As you move to the right, reinforce your lift so that your left hip doesn't drop. Each time you slide left, do your best to maintain the lift on the right side.

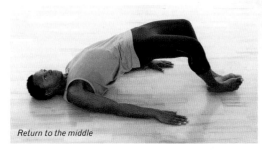

Return to the middle

4. If you wish, purse your lips and breathe out through your mouth, which will help the core muscles to work. Each time you move to the side, the muscles at the side of your waist will activate. After completing eight slow slides, you can work more dynamically. Use a faster exhalation to mirror a strong, quick slide to each side for eight more rounds. Then rest down and hug your knees into your chest.

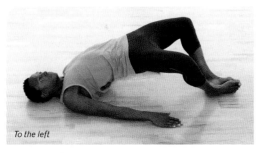

To the left

COBBLER'S BRIDGE

unwind
Blissful Banana (page 286)

take care
Ensure that you have no knee pain during this practice.

banana pose

This is a super-easy pose with a fun name, yet with serious benefits. The relaxing yin-style side-release is profound. Energetically it works on the gall-bladder meridian. Physically it stretches the whole side of the body, the abdominal obliques and the iliotibial band at the outer thigh, which is tight in many people. If you lay yourself out symmetrically after completing one side and test how you feel, you will clearly observe the effects of the pose on your body.

1. Lie on your back with your arms stretched overhead. Take hold of your left wrist with your right hand. Pull on your left wrist a little as you slide your torso into a small right-hand curve. Don't go so far that your left shoulder lifts up. Instead, both shoulder blades will remain with fairly even pressure on the floor.

move forward
Intense Reclining Side-Stretch (page 196)

balance out
Seated Yogic Roll-Downs (page 204)

STRONG, STRETCHY SIDES

2. Next, walk your feet to the right, keeping your left buttock heavy on the floor. Don't go beyond the point where you feel discomfort. Your feet might only move 30–40cm (12–16in). This pose is a case where less is definitely more. To achieve the benefits of it, you will be using the gift of time, rather than an extreme stretch. If it feels good, rest your left ankle on top of your right. Then relax all efforts. Rest here, using soft belly-breathing, for three to five minutes. Set a timer if you like, so that you can be even on each side. Aside from a lovely lengthening along the left side of your body, observe how the right side of your abdomen is pleasantly compressed. Get a sense of the ascending colon on that left side enjoying a squish, like a massage, to help it with its job of digestion. Imagine all the organs on that right side – the liver, gall-bladder and right kidney – getting a yoga massage, to help them with their work of keeping your body healthy. Meanwhile ponder on how all the organs of the left side – the stomach, pancreas, spleen, left kidney and descending colon – experience a soothing and gentle sense of unsquashing, so that they, too, can work really well for your body, to achieve vibrant health.

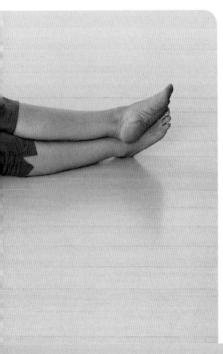

3. Move your legs back to the centre. Then return your upper body to symmetry. As you lie stretched out and floppy, notice how long and relaxed you feel on that left side. Then repeat on the second side.

unwind
Reclining Eagle Twist (page 226)

take care
Seek advice on using this pose if you have sacroiliac dysfunction.

intense reclining side-stretch

This pose is an incredible way to wake up the whole of your side-body. Achieving that final stage requires lots of length in the hamstrings, but read below for a special technique to enable that to occur. Even if you don't quite manage the final stages, you will still get an amazing release, so go ahead and try out this terrific pose.

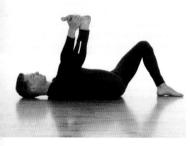

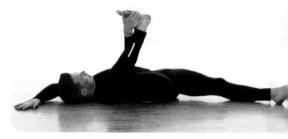

STRONG, STRETCHY SIDES

1. Lie on your back, with your knees bent up and your feet on the floor. Lift your buttocks and move them about 6cm (2½in) to the right. Bend your right knee into your right armpit, then take hold of your right heel in your right hand, to form a half Happy-Baby Pose (see page 158).

2. Now work the right leg straight, in a way that really allows the hamstrings to let go. Press down with your right hand onto your heel, as if to compress the leg bones back into the hip socket. While your hand presses down and your elbow tries to bend, allow your leg to "win": it will straighten as the heel presses away. Once your right leg is as straight as it will go, slide your left foot out to straighten the left leg. Then move that foot about 30cm (12in) to the right, to create a half-banana shape. Finally, drape your left arm along the floor overhead, and slide your hand about 20cm (8in) away to the right, to finish your banana shape. As best you can, rest your torso and left shoulder blade down more heavily on the floor, to enhance this side-stretch.

move forward
Bound Side-Angle Stretch (page 104)

balance out
Yoga Swimming Bow (page 240)

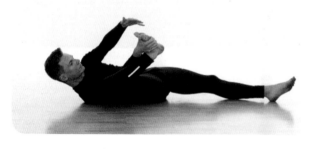

3. To increase the stretch even more, lift your left arm up and across the front of your torso, to catch your right toes with your hand. It helps to lift your head as you do this.

4. Once you have your grip, roll back so that both sides of your back are equally weighted to the floor and rest your head down. Continue to reach away through your right heel. Send energy down through your left leg to your heel as well. Take five to ten long, slow breaths, before coming out to complete side two.

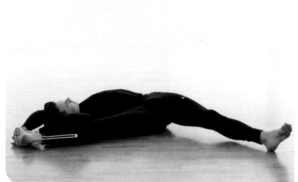

unwind
Corkscrew Twist (page 172)

take care
Take care in cases of sacroiliac dysfunction or if you are at risk of disc herniation.

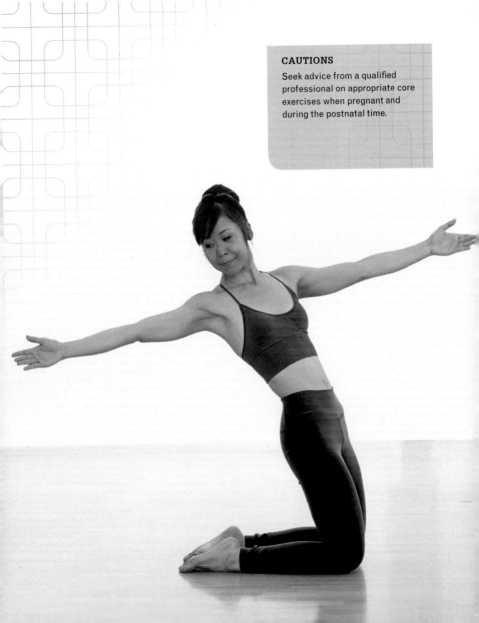

THE JOY OF CORE

Your core is more than just those tummy muscles. Your core muscles include those of the pelvic floor, your back muscles, side-waist muscles and diaphragm. Think of it like a house. You would never build on shaky foundations, so you need to prepare with a strong pelvic floor. You need to build steady walls (belly, side-waist and back) and then a stable roof (diaphragm muscle), too. These muscles work together to give you support and the power to move, and to help you balance. They keep you safe and injury-free.

The core work of classical yoga has become more accessible. Traditionally yoga uses *bandhas*, or energy locks, and the ones that are most relevant to core work are subtle activations of the muscles at the lower abdomen and pelvic floor. The ancient yogis got it right, but these energy locks were tricky to describe in a group yoga class, so not all modern-day yogis could connect with them. Modern-day physiotherapy, plus the influence

of Pilates, has opened the door for today's yogis to develop their core work effectively.

Yoga builds strength by supporting your own weight in a static position, or by organizing you to hold your body correctly as you move. It's lovely to be self-sufficient with your core unity work. No fancy equipment is needed and you can do it anywhere.

While there are core-specific practices in this section, remember that yoga is a great package deal. There are lots more core practices throughout the book to give you core integrity, plus that long-and-lean look. In particular, the planks, inversions and balances build core strength. You will also recruit core muscles doing backbends and working on the side-body. Twists using the core muscles are great, too. If you are new to this type of work, it doesn't take long to notice a significant increase in your core strength, so get started and conquer your core now.

yogic compass

While this excellent starter pose may not seem like the most glamorous of yoga moves, it is essential foundation practice, which ensures that you have a good balance in the working of the various abdominal muscles. Don't skip it – treat it as the valuable investment in your postural health that it is.

1. Lie on your back, with your knees bent up and your feet hip-width apart on the floor. Place your hands flat on your abdomen in a diamond shape, with the tips of your thumb and index finger touching each other. Visualize the hammock of muscles running between your tailbone and your pubic bone – your pelvic-floor muscles.

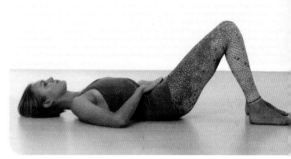

2. Set up a rocking of your pelvis, forward and backward. As you inhale, curve your lower back off the floor as your pelvis tilts posteriorly. Your fingertips will point down and your thumb tips will point up slightly. When you exhale, allow the squeezing of your abdominal muscles to press the lower back down to the floor. Contract the deeper

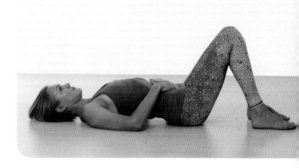

build up
Tiger Flow (page 32)

move forward
Prayer Sweeps (page 206)

balance out
Hip-Releasing Wide Child Pose (page 216)

THE JOY OF CORE

200

layers of the abdominal muscles, so that you feel your belly hollowing down away from your palms. As you perform this scooping-out action, you will also be tucking your tailbone under, and your pelvis will tilt anteriorly. This is a natural time to contract your pelvic-floor muscles and draw this sling of muscles up toward the centre of the torso. When you do this, your fingers will point slightly up and your thumbs will angle down.

3. Continue this slow rocking, as if your abdomen were a compass and you were touching down the North point of it (the tailbone) and the South point (the lowest rib) to the floor. For this entire sequence, move your efforts away from the type of force that makes you furrow your brow or grit your teeth. It's about a softer focus with a happy curiosity, exploring any areas of duller awareness or weaker muscles. Your relaxed breathing rate will be the guiding factor in how slowly you move. Remember: the slower you move, the more you can develop your ability to "scoop". You will also have more time to develop your awareness, and this is key to yoga practice.

4. Now move from your North–South rocking points to explore East and West. First, find the central point that is right in the middle of your North and South. Your lower back will curve gently up from the floor in its natural, neutral arched shape. Then go toward East – contract the abdominal muscles more on your right side, to imprint the right half of your lower back to the floor. Inhale to return to centre, then exhale toward West, working the left half of your belly and focusing on pressing the left lower back to the floor. Mindfully complete ten more East–West moments.

5. Now work clockwise around the compass. First press down the North point, then East, South and West, to return to North. Stay attuned to any lazy parts that won't touch down easily through your circle, and then linger there to build awareness and strength. After five complete rounds, return to the centre and circle anticlockwise five times.

unwind
Expansive Breath Warrior (page 94)

☆ dancing bridge

Cultivate core strength as you move intuitively in a spontaneous, flowing manner. I particularly enjoy this pose, as it reminds me of the innate inner wisdom of my body. It lets me trust that the abdominal muscles will be recruited in just the right way to develop a strong and healthy core. Enjoy the playful, organic feel as you "dance" with your pelvis.

1. Lie on your back and reach your arms up to vertical. As you exhale, lengthen your tailbone away and lift your sacrum up off the floor. Continue to reach away with your tailbone so that your back feels luxuriously long, as you lift your lower back and mid-back up, as high as feels comfortable. Rather than rigidly extending through the elbows, soften them with a gentle bend and allow them to move slightly away from each other. Drop your upper-arm bones into their shoulder sockets, and allow your upper back to broaden and feel heavy on the floor. This will allow you to give yourself a lovely back massage when you begin to move.

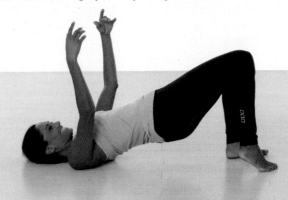

build up
Spine Mobilizer (page 50)

move forward
Core-Activating Plank Flow
(page 212)

balance out
Reclining Eagle Twist (page 226)

THE JOY OF CORE

2. Lift the balls of your feet to swivel your feet to one side, while you sweep your pelvis to the other side, then start to circle the pelvis. Continue to lengthen the tailbone away, so that the lower back doesn't feel compressed. Move away from strict circles, and instead let your pelvis swish and slide. Allow your feet to sway so that they respond in a natural way to your hip movements. Let your arms be guided by the movements of the torso and hips. They may feel like moving in different ways from each other, as they respond to the flowing movements of the pelvis. Go with the flow: make it dance-like. Try out different speeds and directions of movement. Besides the core cultivation, you are also developing hamstring and back muscle strength.

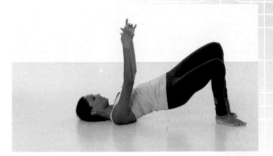

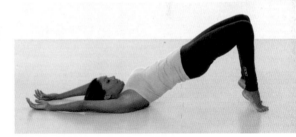

3. To come down in a core-strengthening way, reach your arms overhead along the floor. Lift your heels so your feet are on tiptoes. Tuck your tailbone under to elongate the lower back as much as possible. Touching down from the upper back to the tailbone, lower yourself down. Try to touch each vertebra down one by one. The slower you go, the stronger your workout will be.

DANCING BRIDGE

unwind
Corkscrew Twist (page 172)

take care
Keep your hips fairly low, if taking them any higher creates uncomfortable compression in the lower back.

seated yogic roll-downs

This pose will strengthen the all-important transverse abdominis muscle, which acts like a corset, with its muscle fibres wrapping horizontally around the abdomen. It protects the lower back by switching on as you prepare for movement, and acts as an insurance policy against injury, defending your body from repetitive stressors. It also helps enormously in maintaining good posture.

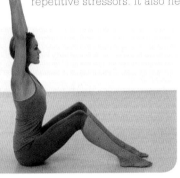

1. Sit with your legs bent in front of you. Have your knees and feet about hip-width apart. Anatomical hip width is often narrower than you might expect: measure it out by placing a fist between your big toes. Inhale and lift your arms overhead as you draw your spine up tall. In particular, pull in the lower back and tilt your pelvis forward as you perform this move.

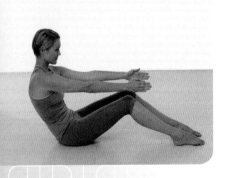

2. As you exhale, draw your navel toward the spine and visualize a hollowing-out of the belly. Reverse your pelvic tilt by tucking your tailbone under. This tuck initiates the rolling down as your spine rounds to a C-shape. As you roll down, lower your arms to horizontal, with the palms on either side of your legs. Inhale as you roll back up and activate your back muscles, to create a long, tall spine. While your arms reach overhead, allow your shoulders to drop down away from your ears. Exhale and scoop at the belly as you roll back down. Repeat for ten or 15 more rounds.

build up	**move forward**	**balance out**
Yogic Compass (page 200)	Dog to Plank Flow (page 210)	Locust Sway (page 234)

3. Now work another two layers of abdominal muscles: the obliques. Inhale as you flatten your back, lift your chest and reach your arms up. When you exhale, roll down and lower both arms to the outer right thigh. Your torso needs to twist only minimally. Most of the sideways movement is done with the arms, and this is enough to engage your rotational oblique muscles. Inhale up to centre, then exhale and roll down, this time with your arms to the left. As you roll down, keep an eye on your abdomen. If it domes outward, the wrong muscles are working. Don't roll down as far, so that you can ensure it hollows inward while you develop strength. Complete ten more rounds, alternating sides.

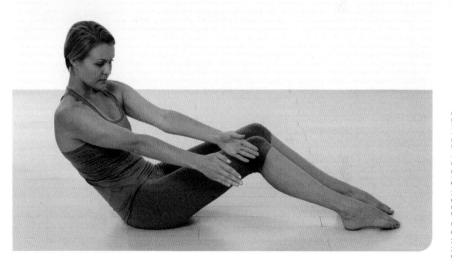

unwind
Blissful Banana (page 286)

take care
If you are losing your alignment, keep your hands on your thighs to make it easier. Work with an experienced teacher to modify your core strength work during pregnancy. Don't round the spine if you have a recent or chronic disc injury.

☆ prayer sweeps

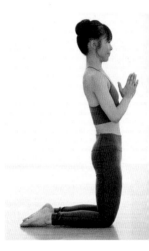

This sequence is great at working the deepest three layers of the four layers of the abdominal muscles. It's the yoga way to avoid feeling as if you need shapewear, as it keeps your waist looking trim.

1. Come into a high kneeling position and bring your palms together at the heart centre. Observe the natural curves of your spine in this starting point. Then tuck your tailbone under and feel your lower abdominal muscles activate. It helps to exhale as you do this action. Cultivate the activation of the pelvic-floor muscles at the same time as each exhalation. Inhale and allow your spine to return to its normal curves, then exhale again to tilt your pelvis forward. As you do this, you will feel the beginnings of a stretch through the front of your thighs. When your deeper core muscles are working, your waist draws in to become more slender.

2. Once you have completed several tucking-under rounds, add on a lean-back with your torso as you exhale. Don't allow your ribcage to open in the front as you move back. Instead, melt the lower front ribs down into the upper abdomen, feeling your upper belly firm. Aim to create a straight line from your knees, through the hips to your shoulders. You might feel a good stretch through the front thighs, too. Complete five rounds.

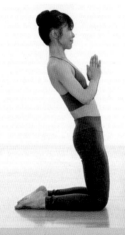

THE JOY OF CORE

build up	**move forward**	**balance out**
Flying Locust (page 38)	Hip-Freeing Dog to Plank (page 66)	Hip-Releasing Wide Child Pose (page 216)

3. Next time you inhale, return to your upright starting point and reach both arms out in front, roughly horizontal. As you exhale, release your right arm down and move it through a low arc to reach back. Keep both shoulders soft as you reach away. Inhale to return your right arm in front, palms facing each other and elbows softy bent. Exhale, lift your pelvic-floor muscles, lean back and rotate to the left, with your eyes following the moving thumb. Then inhale and return to the centre. Alternating sides, continue for eight more rounds.

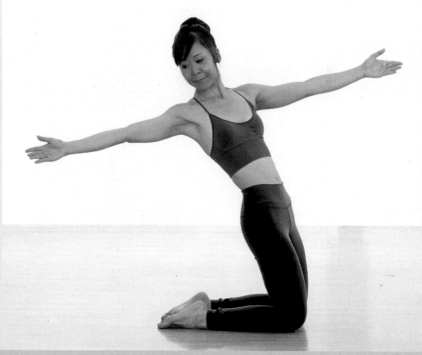

unwind
Kinky Cobbler's Pose
(page 154)

take care
Kneel on a soft blanket if your knees require padding.

plough-pose lifts

This pose is great for targeting the lower abdominals in particular, and is a really nice one for bringing flexibility and ease to the lower back. Each time you roll down slowly it's like a massage for those tight lower-back muscles. This is great preparation for coming into and out of Basic Shoulder-Stand (see page 258).

1. Lie on your back and bend your knees up to bring your feet in the air. Place your index fingers into the creases behind your knees. As you exhale, use your abdominal muscles to lift your sacrum off the floor. Your elbows will bend and widen as you lift. As you breathe in, roll your back down to the floor again. It will be a fairly fast movement as you roll up and down. Your hips can flex, so that your knees will move forward as you lift up. Then let the knees move away from you as you roll down, and allow your elbows to straighten. If your lower back feels stiff and clunky, try using soft padding underneath and take only tiny movements. If it still doesn't feel good, or feels too explosive for your comfort, practise Prayer Sweeps (see page 206) instead.

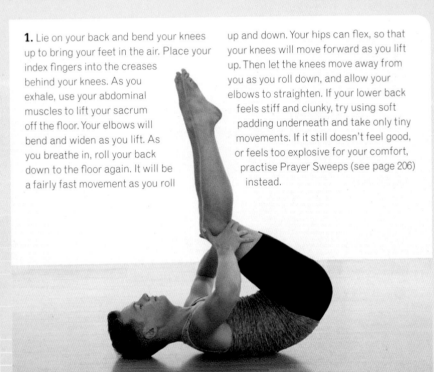

build up
Tiger Flow (page 32)

move forward
Basic Shoulder-Stand
(page 258)

balance out
Bow Pose Three Ways
(page 238)

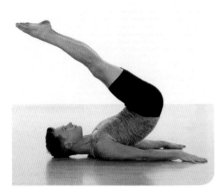

2. Now slow the movement down, to build on your core control. Lengthen your arms along the floor, palms down. Pressing down with the palms, inhale and lift up your sacrum, possibly lifting the hips higher this time and working a little further up the spine. If you feel strong in your core and flexible in your forward bends, you will be able to work with straight legs, as shown; but if you need to bend the knees, that works well, too.

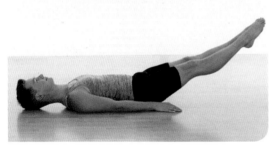

3. Now start to roll back down, using your palms against the floor to help slow this movement down. Exhale, draw your navel toward the spine and take your legs slightly away from vertical. Each time you repeat, take your legs a little further toward the floor. If you are unable to scoop your belly in, that's a sign you have gone too far: either bend your knees or don't lower so far, or both. Most people keep their legs closer to vertical than horizontal in this practice. The aim is not to have your legs hovering above the floor, which is super-difficult. It's more important that your core works correctly here than insist on large movements. Complete ten rounds, then rest.

unwind
Reclining Eagle Twist
(page 226)

take care
Avoid this pose during menstruation, pregnancy or if you suffer from lower-back conditions, such as disc herniation.

dog to plank flow

This is great all-over core work. The rippling effect builds integrity by working the deeper core layers, while the Plank action will strengthen the rectus abdominis – that handsome muscle otherwise known as the "six-pack", which features so heavily on the covers of fitness magazines.

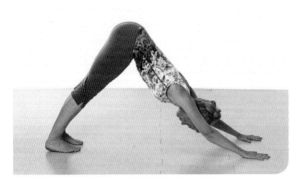

1. Start in Classic Downward-Facing Dog Pose (see page 58). To get started on the pelvic-tilt action, bend your knees and lift up onto tiptoes. Now tuck your tailbone under to a pelvic tilt. You will feel your lower back lengthening out and your abdominal muscles squeezing. Throughout this sequence you can continue to initiate the pelvic rotation with bent knees, if you have tighter hamstrings; but if your hamstrings are quite flexible, try it out with straight legs, as shown.

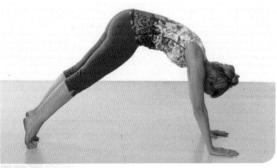

THE JOY OF CORE

build up	**move forward**	**balance out**
Seated Yogic Roll-Downs (page 204)	Inclined Plane Pose (page 190)	Pigeon Limbering (page 54)

2. Move your hips forward into the Plank position, with shoulders over wrists. As you come into this pose, move from your hips first and finish at your neck. You'll create a ripple-like action as you move from bottom to top. It might help to mentally divide your spine into small segments of a few vertebrae each. Assisted by the abdominal muscles, each vertebral chunk will briefly lift toward the sky, even as your overall shape lowers to form the straight line of a plank. Perform this action on an inhalation and breathe slowly, so that you have plenty of time.

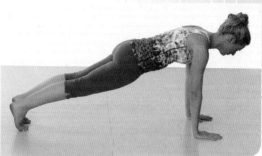

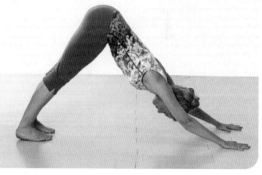

3. Once you are in the Plank position, exhale and lift your navel away from the ground. With the abdominals firmly drawing in, take your hips up and back into Downward-Facing Dog once again. Allow for a nice long, slow exhalation, so that your heels have time to ease down toward the floor for a good calf stretch.

4. Now set up your flowing movement, the speed of which will be guided by your breath. Inhaling, tilt your pelvis backward and ripple the movement up your spine into the Plank position. Exhale, squeeze on the abdominals and move to Downward-Facing Dog. Repeat six to ten times, then rest.

DOG TO PLANK FLOW

unwind
Resting Cobbler's Poses (page 284)

take care
The full Plank should not be practised when pregnant or during the post-natal period. If your wrists are sore, you can do a similar practice facing a wall, with your hands on the wall and your feet stepped back.

core-activating plank flow

Use the reliability of the flow to encourage you throughout this challenging sequence. As you linger in the three Plank positions, have faith that before long, the next inhalation will sweep you up and away to the next nice, stretchy Dog Pose. An easier version is to stay on hands and knees.

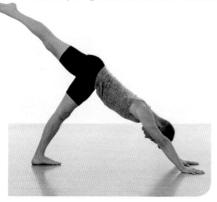

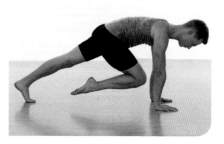

1. From the Classic Downward-Facing Dog Pose (see page 58), inhale and lift your right leg into a high Dog Split. Press down through both palms and reach away through the ball of the right foot.

2. Exhale to start to move your torso forward to a Plank position, with shoulders above wrists. As you do so, bend your right knee into the breastbone, as if you wanted to kiss it. Lift your abdomen strongly up and away from the earth. At the same time lift your chest, so that your thoracic spine rounds upward. As you lift your vertebrae, allow your shoulder blades to spread, and press down firmly through the fingertips.

THE JOY OF CORE

build up
Tiger Flow (page 32)

move forward
Strengthening Sun Salutation (page 76)

balance out
Gate Pose with Side Bow (see page 44)

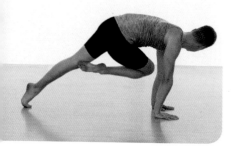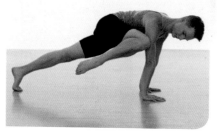

3. Exhale and, moving with a strong core focus, send your right leg back and up as you take your hips into the Dog Split. Inhale, suck in the abdominals again and return to the Plank position, this time with your right knee moving toward your left armpit, so that you create a rotation and enhance your oblique muscle strength.

4. Exhale, keep your abdominals engaged and lift back up to Dog Split. On your next inhalation, come forward to the Plank position once again, this time taking your right knee wide to the outer upper arm on the right side. Exhale to return to your Dog Split, then lower your right foot down. Rest, and circle your wrists to ease them. Then practise the second side.

unwind
Wide-Legged Spirals
(page 220)

take care
The full Plank position should not be practised when pregnant, or during the post-natal period.

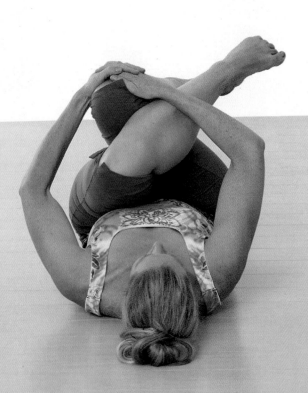

11

HAPPY HIPS

If there is anything guaranteed to have you feeling slinky and supple as you walk – or sashay – out of yoga class, it's a good hip-releasing sequence.

Being ball-and-socket joints, your hips have an amazing range of motion, but if you have a sedentary lifestyle, you might not be fully utilizing their capabilities. If your daily life involves lots of desk-time during work hours, slouched couch-time after work and seated commuter-time in between, then this could be the most life-enhancing section for you.

Hip stretches can help correct spine and pelvic misalignments, and relieve back pain, soreness and general stiffness. Aim to stretch all around your hip joint by practising some wide-legged inner-thigh stretches and lunging-style releases for the fronts of your hips, and by releasing those tight rotator muscles at the buttocks and outer hips.

There are plenty of other gorgeous hip releases throughout this book: do be sure to check out the "Yin Yoga" section, too (see pages 304–27), for some stunners. With lots of tissue layers around the hips, you want to take a little time, so don't rush through the poses. Stay for at least a minute in each one. Linger and love the lusciousness of feeling light, free and floaty.

☆ hip-releasing wide child pose

There are so many layers of muscle and fascia around the hips it's understandable that getting them to release requires a little time in the postures. The restful nature of this pose gives your hips just the time they need. More than simply a hip-opener, this version of the Child Pose stretches the shoulders and elongates the torso, too. Do take this delicious opportunity to settle into the pose and sink into enjoyment, while you soften and stretch out.

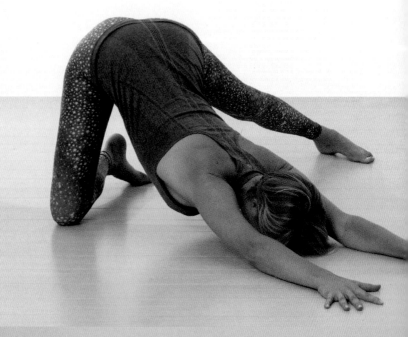

build up
Spine-Mobilizing Lunge
(page 42)

move forward
Power Squat (page 218)

balance out
Cow-Pose Spirals (page 222)

1. Start on all fours. Move your right knee wide, to point out to the right, and bring your right toes to the centre, in line with your tailbone.

2. Take your left leg out to the left. Position your left foot so that both heels are in one line. Arrange your left foot mindfully. Have all your left toes pointing forward. Now focus on pressing down evenly on all four corners of your foot: the big-toe knuckle, the little-toe knuckle, the inner-heel edge and the outer-heel edge. Resist the urge to roll your foot in, collapsing the inner arch. Instead, enliven the workings of your foot and keep your inner arch lifted. Come down onto your forearms with your hips in the air. If possible, slide your left foot further to the left to find a satisfying and manageable stretch along the inner thigh.

3. Keeping your buttocks high in the air and roughly in line with both heels, walk your hands forward and allow the heart centre to open toward the floor. Rest your forehead on the floor and, with palms placed as far forward as possible, lift both elbows. Enjoy the sensations of length in your torso and of release in your shoulders. Think of dropping your armpits down lower, while energizing your elbows so that they lift higher. Just as in the Classic Downward-Facing Dog Pose (see page 58), press all the knuckles of your fingers and thumbs evenly into the floor. Stay for five to 15 long, smooth breaths. Then come out, ready for side two.

unwind
Pigeon Limbering (page 54)

take care
This pose can feel lovely until 35 weeks during pregnancy, but avoid it during the post-natal phrase. Avoid inversions if you suffer from high blood pressure, eye issues such as a detached retina or a risk of glaucoma.

power squat

☆
☆
☆

This martial-arts-inspired sequence brings power to the thighs, while the stretch works into the hips and inner thighs. It strengthens the muscles around the knees, which can help in a range of knee problems.

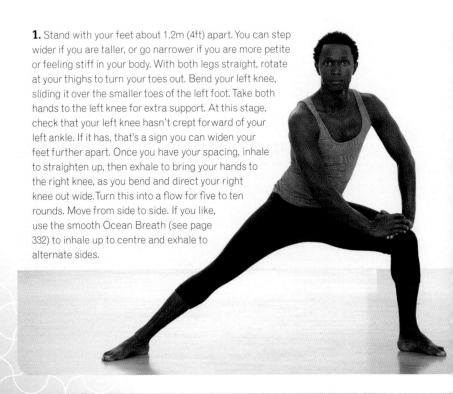

1. Stand with your feet about 1.2m (4ft) apart. You can step wider if you are taller, or go narrower if you are more petite or feeling stiff in your body. With both legs straight, rotate at your thighs to turn your toes out. Bend your left knee, sliding it over the smaller toes of the left foot. Take both hands to the left knee for extra support. At this stage, check that your left knee hasn't crept forward of your left ankle. If it has, that's a sign you can widen your feet further apart. Once you have your spacing, inhale to straighten up, then exhale to bring your hands to the right knee, as you bend and direct your right knee out wide. Turn this into a flow for five to ten rounds. Move from side to side. If you like, use the smooth Ocean Breath (see page 332) to inhale up to centre and exhale to alternate sides.

build up	**move forward**	**balance out**
Hip-Releasing Wide Child Pose (page 216)	Yin Frog (page 324)	Shoulder-Releasing Eagle (page 116)

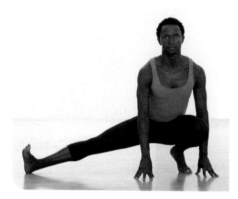 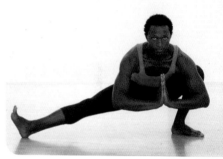

2. Once you feel warmed up, and if your knees are feeling good, take it a little lower and deeper. Bring your fingers to the floor as you drop your seat down, aiming for your left sitting bone to hover above your left heel. Lift your left heel. On the right side, lift your toes and press the heel of the right foot away to increase the inner-thigh stretch. While easing into this hip-opening action, firm the back muscles along the spine. This will help you to lift your torso up as tall as possible.

3. Once you have the upward lift in the torso, join the palms together in prayer and, once again, draw yourself upright so that you feel as tall as possible. You may be able to drop your left heel to the floor. Exhale away any tightness in the hips or inner right thigh. After five long, round breaths, draw up your pelvic-floor muscles and use the strength in your legs to come up and move into the right side.

unwind
Reclining Eagle Twist
(page 226)

take care
Work within the limits of your knees and never go where there is pain.

wide-legged spirals

Time and again this practice reminds me of how working gently, with
a reliable rhythm, encourages the body to feel safe enough to surrender
its tensions. The smooth spiralling enables the pelvic and thigh areas
to soften, but more than that happens: it's almost as if the brain itself
softens into a hypnotic space and your thoughts are soothed.

1. Sit with your legs stretched out wide.
Bend your knees up a little, to allow your
pelvis to tilt forward enough to enable
you to sit up tall with less effort. Notice
how the most central part of your two
sitting bones connects with the earth.
Begin to circle your torso above your
hips. Sway to the right side of your
sitting bones, then move slowly
forward, so that you feel
yourself on the

front edges of your sitting bones. Continue
your circle left and lean back a little, to
start to involve your abdominal muscles
more. Continue to move in larger and larger
circles, until you feel that your arms want
to get involved, too. Reach your hands out
to one side as you sway to that side,
then in front as you move forward.
Each time you lean back, bend the
elbows to bring your hands
closer to your chest.

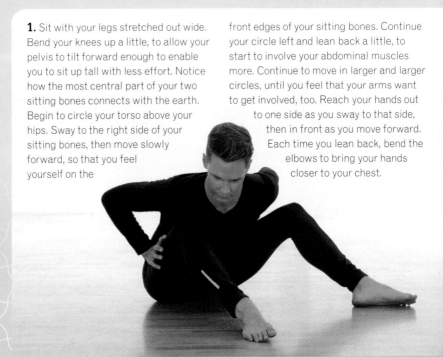

build up
Seaweed Sway (page 106)

move forward
Standing Splits (page 122)

balance out
Locust Sway (page 234)

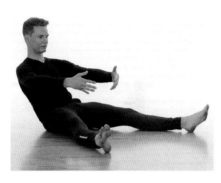

2. Once the circling has freed up your pelvis somewhat, straighten your legs and continue in ever-increasing spirals. If you are very flexible and want more anchoring, reach the heels away and press the backs of your knees to the floor. Ensure that you lean well into the back of your circle, to engage your core muscles.

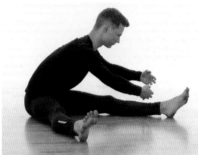

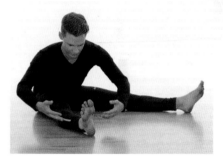

3. After ten or more spirals, change direction. This time start off with your largest circles. After a few generous circles with no flat edges, reduce the circumference bit by bit. Move in smaller and smaller spirals until, after many rounds, you find yourself sitting still. Rest your hands on your thighs. Once you have found your still centre, above

the axis of your pelvis, notice how your torso lifts and your posture may feel long and dignified. While your outer body is now in stillness, notice how your inner body may still feel a little swirly. Your brain might even feel more relaxed by now. Relax into these sensations as you enjoy your breathing for a little longer here.

unwind
Slinky Shoulders, Gleeful
Glutes (page 142)

take care
Ensure that you protect your back in all forward bends
if you are at risk of a slipped disc.

cow-pose spirals

Here we combine two classic poses: we take the legs of Cow-Face Pose, for a gluteal and outer-hip release, and add the shoulder-releasing arms of Intense Forward Stretch. Add some preliminary loosening movements to a long, deep release, and you will dissolve away your creaks and squeaks.

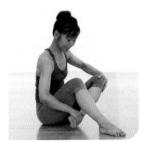

1. Sit on the floor with your legs bent up in front. Reach your right hand under your right thigh to take hold of your left ankle. Pull your foot through to rest by your right outer hip. Grasp your right ankle in your left hand and lift that leg up and over, to position your right foot near your left outer hip. As best you can, stack your right knee on top of your left knee. If that's not possible for you, stretch out your left leg in front and position the right leg on top, with the foot near the left outer hip and the knees stacked as much as possible.

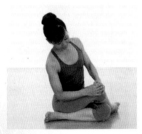 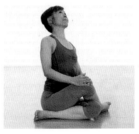 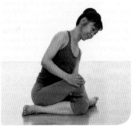

2. Interlace your fingers to cup your top knee. Start to circle your torso above your hips – find a speed that feels nice. While it appears externally that your hips don't move, as you circle, become pleasantly aware of the various lines of stretch that you feel. Let the circling action dissolve the tensions bit by bit. After eight or more rounds, circle the other way. Notice any tight spots and how much they, too, release.

HAPPY HIPS

build up
Hip-Freeing Dog to Plank
(page 66)

move forward
Revolved Bound Lunge
(page 92)

balance out
Heavenly Happy-Baby Pose
(page 158)

3. Come to stillness. Take both arms out wide and, rotating from the shoulders, turn your thumbs forward and down and back. Bring your palms together behind your back in reverse prayer. If you can't get your fingers to point up, have them pointing down. It's easier still to hold each forearm with the opposite hand. Inhale and draw yourself up tall. Then exhale and, folding from the hips, tip forward. First, aim to close the gap between your belly and thigh. Next, reach your heart centre beyond the top knee – imagine your heart is full of runny honey, and aim to drizzle it over the front of the knee. Create a line of energy from your tailbone along the spine and out through the crown of your head. With your right leg on top, you'll feel the main stretch in the right buttock. Hold for eight full, deep breaths. Then repeat on the other side.

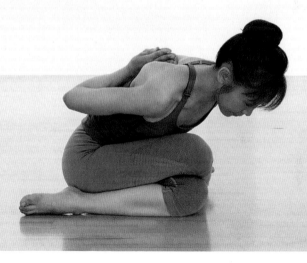

unwind
Resting Cobbler's Poses
(page 284)

take care
Seek advice if you have shoulder or hip injuries.

☆ pigeon pose with scientific stretching
☆

This scientific stretching technique works a treat for your hips in Pigeon Pose. You get a lot of stretch in a short time by using the technique of PNF stretching, otherwise known as "proprioceptive neuromuscular facilitation". The same contract-then-release technique that you will try here can be applied to many other yoga stretches.

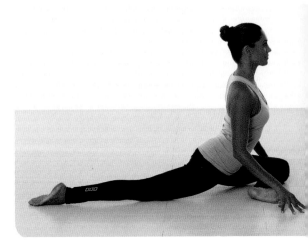

1. From an all-fours position, slide your left knee forward to your left wrist. Move your left foot toward your right wrist. Now slide your right leg straight back as your hips lower toward the floor. Square your hips off as much as possible, by easing the right hip forward. Curve your spine into a long, sloping backbend. This is your starter Pigeon Pose. If you are fairly flexible, ease your left knee further to the left and edge your left foot further forward. Your right foot and knee may even be in one line. Continue to press your right hip forward. If your hips are tighter, position your front leg so that your your knee is further forward than your front foot.

build up	**move forward**	**balance out**
Pigeon Limbering (page 54)	Pigeon Crescent Pose (page 242)	Spine-Mobilizing Lunge (page 42)

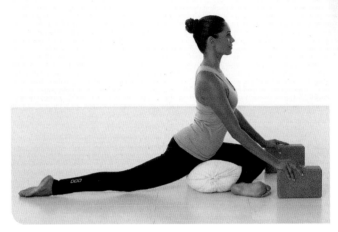

muscle power
and contract for
six seconds. Your
basic position
won't change,
but your hips will
float up slightly.
Then release the
contraction and,

2. If you experience knee pain, try using the support of a bolster or folded blankets under the front thigh, to lift the hip higher than your knee. It can be helpful to place each hand on a yoga brick, too. If you still have knee pain, discontinue this pose. If you are comfortable, move into the active assisted stretch. Keep both knees on the floor, yet contract your muscles as if trying to slide your back knee forward and your front knee backward. Use about 30 per cent of your

on an exhale, soften everything, allow your hips to drop and slide your back leg further away. Hold the stretch for 30 seconds, then reduce the intensity to rest for 30 seconds. Once again, contract your muscles at only 30 per cent intensity, as if to slide your knees toward each other, for six seconds, then release. Slide your legs away, to stretch into the left buttock and the front of the right hip for 30 seconds. Then use your hands to help you come out, ready for the second side.

unwind
Head-Beyond-the-Knee Pose
(page 160)

take care
Protect vulnerable knees by keeping your hip joint higher than your knee joint in this pose. Discontinue if there is any discomfort. Lean forward more if you feel discomfort in the lower back.

☆ reclining eagle twist
☆

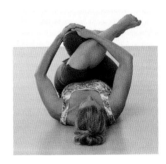

What's not to love about this sequence? You'll get a release of tension in the hips and outer thighs from the leg positioning. Your back will get a great stretch due to the twisting action, plus all that good energy flow that goes with it. And all while being a little lazy, as you get to lie down.

1. Lie on your back and bring your legs into the air. With both knees bent, cross your left thigh in front of your right thigh. Take your hands to the top shin and hug both knees in, for five or more long breaths.

2. Keeping your legs crossed, take your feet to the floor. Lift your buttocks off the floor, to move your hips 5cm (2in) to the left side. Then lift your legs and use your abdominals to bring your thighs in as close as possible to your torso. With arms spread wide, lower your legs to the right. If the floor feels too far away for comfort, place cushions underneath, so that the stretch on the lower back is not as intense. Choose a comfortable position for your neck. You may prefer looking right, up, left or anywhere in between. Stay for eight or more breaths.

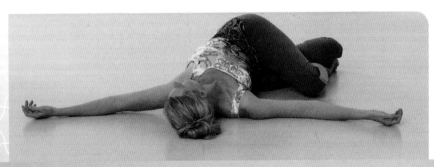

build up
Shoulder-Releasing Eagle (page 116)

move forward
Shoelace (page 316)

balance out
Yin Happy Baby (page 318)

3. To come up safely, unwrap your legs and bring them up one by one. Then wrap them up the same way as before, left thigh on top of right. Take your feet to the floor, lift your hips to move them 10cm (4in) to the right (so that you have returned to spinal symmetry and then moved 5cm/2in to the right of that centre position). Draw the thighs in again, raising your feet into the air, and then lower them to the left side. This side will be more challenging, so be open to taking some support under the legs on this side. Relax into this position as you broaden across the upper back and soften your right shoulder to the floor. Settle on a good position for your neck, ensuring it feels comfortable. Stay for eight breaths or more. Unravel your legs to come up. Practise the second side, with your right thigh stacked on top of the left.

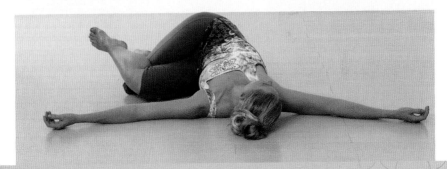

unwind
Blissful Banana
(page 286)

take care
If your lower back is vulnerable, do place some support under the legs to lift them.

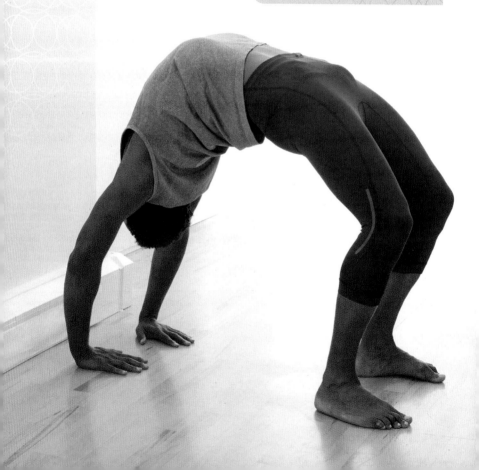

12

BLISSFUL BACKBENDS

Energizing, rejuvenating, invigorating, uplifting, revitalizing – backbends offer all of these wonderful things. The list sounds like a magic elixir that we wish we could bottle. We can't bottle it to sell, but the good news is that backbends are within your grasp, if you are willing to put in the time.

We all need a balance between suppleness and strength. Some backbends are stretch-based, while others are more strength-based. Despite their caffeine-like boosting effects, backbends are not like that favourite coffee you are stuck on – a little variety is good. When choosing your backbend blend for the day, it is vital to practise at least one that strengthens the muscles, as well as another that targets flexibility.

Backbends undo the generalized slouching and hunching of our modern-day, desk-based, TV-binging, commuter and computer-bound lives. They are important for good posture and more. Energetically, backbends elevate the chest and allow us to greet the world with an open heart. And isn't that what our world needs so badly?

☆ shoulder-loving cobra

I find that my young children benefit from time spent alone with their mummy. Each requires this dedicated, just-for-herself love and support to blossom and grow. So what I love about this practice is that it allows me to spend one-on-one time with each shoulder. It reminds me never to underestimate the power of spending dedicated time connecting with individual part of the body – particularly those sore, tight or injured bits. Terrific breakthroughs and great healing can occur when you give these parts your undivided attention.

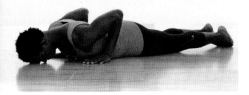 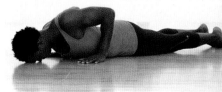

1. Lie on your front, with your hands palms down under the shoulders. Line up your fingertips with the tops of your shoulders. With your fingers spread apart, your longest finger will point straight ahead. However, if you have muscly or stiff shoulders, you may like to swivel the palms out, so that your index fingers point forward. Your elbows will be in the air. Rather than allowing them to splay apart, draw them toward each other, as if they were long-lost lovers.

2. Turn your attention to your left shoulder. In a large circular action, drop your shoulder down, move it forward and up toward your left ear, then complete the circle back and down, drawing your left shoulder blade toward the waist. Your left shoulder will now be lifted higher and will be nicely set back, compared to your right.

build up
Shoulder Sweeps (page 34)

move forward
Three-Up Bridge Pose
(page 246)

balance out
Yin Shoulder Stretches
(page 322)

BLISSFUL BACKBENDS

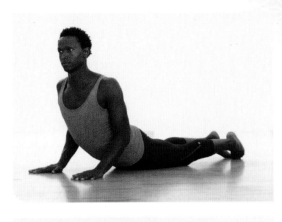

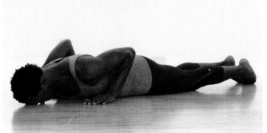

3. On your next inhalation, press through both palms to lift your chest into Cobra Pose. Keep your elbows bent. On an exhalation, lower down, forehead to the floor. Now focus on your right shoulder. Inhale to circle it forward, up, back and down, letting the shoulder blade glide down over the back of the ribs. On the same inhalation, lift up into Cobra, keeping the back of your neck long. Exhale to slowly lower down. Return to your first shoulder, inhaling as you first circle it, then lift. Exhale down. Continue for several more rounds, alternating shoulders as you lift on your inhalations and lower on your exhalations. Enjoy your shoulder joints softening and opening.

4. To finish, work symmetrically. From the low position, roll both shoulders back and down, then draw the bottom edges of your shoulder blades toward each other. Reach out through the crown of the head as you move your chestbone forward and lift up to your Cobra. Hold for five to ten breaths. Then lower down to rest.

unwind
Heavenly Happy-Baby Pose
(page 158)

take care
If you feel discomfort in the lower back, reduce any compression by pushing the pubic bone into the floor before you lift up, and don't lift so high. Don't practise this after ten weeks of pregnancy.

☆ japanese back-strengthener

This super-strengthening back work is adapted from Ryoho, a type of Japanese yoga. It's energizing, powerful and fun, and the breathing-out through the mouth is really helpful in this strengthening work. The connection between the forehead and the hands means that your neck will maintain a healthy alignment, too.

1. Lie face-down and make a pillow with your hands, with one flat on top of the other, palms down. Place your forehead on your hands. Make sure you can breathe through your nose comfortably, by drawing your chin in.

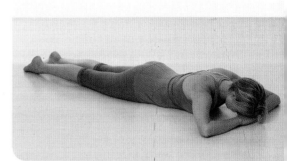

2. Prepare for the lift-up by anchoring your pubic bone to the floor in a slight pelvic-tilt action. Draw your navel into your body, as if to lighten the weight of your abdomen on the floor. Press the tops of your feet to the floor. Firm your kneecaps to create super-straight legs, and energize just the kneecaps away from the floor. Now you are ready to inhale and lift up your chest and arms. Keep your forehead touching your top hand to maintain the length in the back of the neck.

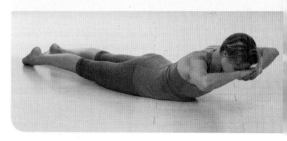

build up
Flying Locust (page 38)

move forward
Half-Frog, Half-Locust (page 236)

balance out
Revolved Happy Pose (page 174)

BLISSFUL BACKBENDS

3. As you exhale through the mouth, curve your spine to the right as you sweep your upper body to that side. Reinforce your lift, to keep an even height through each side. Resist lowering the side that you sway toward. Inhale through your nose to return to centre, then exhale and glide your upper body to the left. Continue for ten more rounds, inhaling to centre and exhaling to alternate sides. Once you find your flow, and if your back is feeling good, speed up a bit. Make your exhalations strong and fairly fast, and allow each sideways sway to reflect that, too, so that they become strong, firm and focused movements that build heat in your back. As you breathe and glide, maintain the anchoring-down of the pubic bone and feet. At the same time, draw your kneecaps and your abdomen away from the floor.

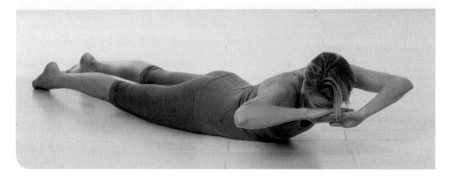

unwind
Wide-Legged Spirals
(page 220)

take care
If you are lacking in strength, keep your fingertips to the floor in front and practise a lighter swaying movement.

☆ locust sway

Part of the trick in developing backbends is to allow the front of the body to stretch and lengthen. This paves the way for the spine to achieve a lovely long and comfortable curve. This Locust variation encourages the front-body release that you need in order to develop flexibility in your backbends, plus there's a nice little twisting action for good measure.

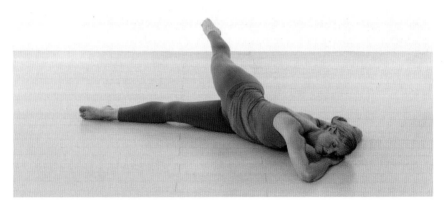

1. Lie on your front and, making a pillow with the backs of your hands, turn your head to the right. Slide your right foot away a little, then lift your right leg up in the air. Keep extending out along the length of the leg to the toes, as you lift your right hip and sway your raised leg to the left. Lifting the right hip will allow your hips to stack, one on top of the other. Keep your raised leg roughly parallel to the floor. While you enjoy five to ten steady breaths in this position, develop a radiation of energies out through the right elbow. With a squeezing action, slide your elbow wider to the right and further forward. You might enjoy a pleasant sense of release in the abdomen. Once you have finished, come out and practise the second side.

build up	**move forward**	**balance out**
Japanese Back-Strengthener (page 232)	Pigeon Crescent Pose (page 242)	Sage Pose with Neck Releases (page 176)

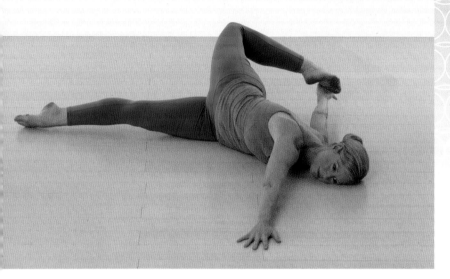

2. Now straighten your arms out wide, palms down and level with your shoulders. Turn your face to the right. Again slide your right leg away, then lift it up and sway it over to the left. Once again, stack your right hip above the left. Now bend your right knee and see if you can catch your right foot in your left hand. Press your foot against your hand so that it moves away from your buttocks, to increase the backbend. Use your hand to guide the back foot up toward the line of your shoulders, too. At the same, time deepen the backbend by "anchoring" yourself more – press your right hip forward, to help open more through the front of the right thigh. Stay for five to ten breaths. Then repeat on the second side.

unwind
Three-Step Reclining Twist
(page 170)

take care
Take extra care if you have facet-joint issues. Never work into discomfort. Don't practise this pose after ten weeks of pregnancy.

half-frog, half-locust

This pose combines the Locust Pose on one side and the Frog Pose on the other. While it develops flexibility on one side, it builds strength and length on the other. This reduces any tendency to over-compression, and the benefits are far-reaching – despite the half-and-half name of this pose, there is certainly no dilution of the benefits of the backbends here. The elements of this pose have a great synergy together, and the benefits definitely add up to more than the sum of their parts.

1. Lie on your front, with your arms stretched forward and shoulder-width apart. Rest your forehead on the floor and magnetize your chin toward your throat, to ensure you can easily breathe through your nose. To come into the Half-Frog Pose, bend your right knee and reach back with your right hand to grasp the front of the foot. Ease your heel toward your buttock and, if it touches, move the foot to the side to allow the right heel to scrape past the right hip toward the floor.

Lowering the heel will occur best if the right buttock is relaxed, so soften it as much as possible. As backbends usually require the activation of the buttocks, it can take a little practice to allow these muscles to release. Once the right foot drops low enough, you may be able to swivel on the heel of the hand so that the right fingers first move out to the right and then point forward, as shown in step 2. This will give a good stretch through the front of the shoulder.

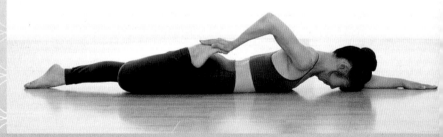

build up
East–West Flow (page 48)

move forward
Dancer's Bow (page 124)

balance out
Threaded Needle (page 180)

2. Now enliven the left half of your body with Half-Locust Pose. Press the top of the left foot down onto the floor. Lift your left kneecap off the floor as you activate the muscles around the knee to keep it straight. Squeezing on the

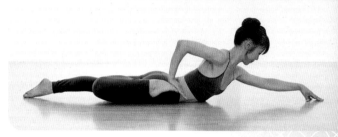

muscles of the back, lift up your chest. Let your left hand slide toward you, as the chest, shoulder and elbow lift away from the floor. Rather than placing any pressure on the left hand, ensure that all the hard work is being done with your back and the anchoring left-leg muscles. Maintain the sense that you could lift your left hand in the air without causing your chest to drop.

3. Stay for a few breaths, appreciating the half-and-half nature of the pose – right side fairly relaxed, left side working hard. Then increase the challenge by lifting your left leg in the air, reaching it away as if to make space in the hip

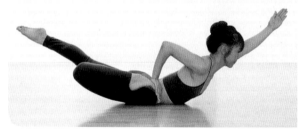

joint. Turn your left thumb upward and lift your left arm up, too. While the left arm reaches away, keep the shoulder blade drawing toward the waist, so that you don't hunch. While your left side is strong, your right side still has a softer energy to it, continuing to allow the right heel to ease downward. Hold for five deliberate and focused breaths. Then practise the second side.

HALF-FROG, HALF-LOCUST

---

unwind
Starter Headstand (page 264)

take care
If your bent knee hurts in the Frog Pose, push the foot away from you to work with a straight arm in Half-Bow Pose (page 238) instead. Avoid this pose during pregnancy.

bow pose three ways

The Bow Pose holds a special place in my heart. Where sometimes yoga students might experience a backbend as a bit too squishy in the lower back, they often find the Bow Pose acceptable and can work into it with gusto. In this version, as the hands change position, a new dimension is added with the shoulder stretches. This allows you to ease a little deeper, with the uplifting and heart-opening movements of the classic Bow.

1. Start by lying face-down on your mat. Reach back to grasp your ankles. Roll your shoulders back, then inhale and press your legs away as you lift your chest away from the floor. As well as pressing back and away with your feet, lift them high. Create the largest possible pocket of air between your back and legs. Press your chestbone forward and up. Allow your belly to feel soft. Create a long, full roundness along the front of your body and allow your chest to lift high. If you are more flexible, you may experience a natural rock forward on each exhale and backward on each inhale. Enjoy the movements over five to ten long breaths.

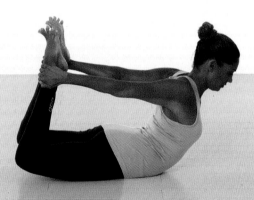

build up
Strengthening Sun Salutation
(page 76)

move forward
One-Legged Upward-Facing
Bow (page 248)

balance out
Bound Side-Angle Stretch
(page 104)

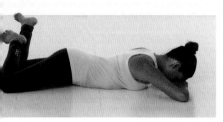

2. Come down and rest your forehead on the pillow of your hands. Bend your knees so that your feet sit above your knees, then sway your feet both to the right, then both to the left a few times, like windscreen wipers. If you can't move on to the next stages, repeat the first stage twice more, as each repetition should feel better.

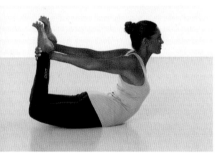

3. Prepare to come up again. This time wrap your right hand around the inside of your right ankle and grasp your left inner ankle with your left hand. Inhale to lift up and enjoy the broadening of the collar bones and the enhanced roll-back of the shoulders. Hold for five to ten breaths once again. Then rest down.

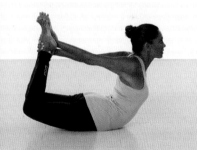

4. For the final stage, reach your arms back and, crossing at your wrists, swap ankles. Hold your right inner ankle in your left hand and your left inner ankle in your right. Ensure that you have actually crossed over at your wrists rather than your ankles. Each time your breathe in, feel the expansion of your ribcage and soar skyward; each time you breathe out, allow the abdomen to soften and relax. After five to ten breaths come down and rest.

unwind
Shoulder-Releasing Forward Fold (page 108)

take care
Any pain is your body telling you that something is wrong, so never hold a pose where you feel pain.

BOW POSE THREE WAYS

☆ yoga swimming bow

This is a great way to build muscle power and warmth in the back muscles. As you stretch gloriously long and lift against gravity, you are getting some strong and healthy postural work. It's also very

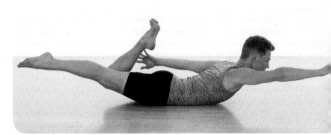

safe, as you are using your own muscle power to lift against gravity, so over-enthusiastic yogis are protected from overdoing it with their backbend.

1. Start by lying on your front with your elbows bent toward your waist. Tuck your tailbone under slightly, to lengthen the lower back. Lift your abdomen away from the floor. You might like to imagine that you are a belly dancer, with a large colourful gem in your navel. Lift your precious stone away from the floor and at the same time press your pubic bone down to the floor.

2. Lift your legs up and reach them back and away. Lift your chest and get ready to free-flow. Try bending one knee to lift your toes while you reach forward with the opposite arm, then move your limbs the other way, so that your movements become a dance. In turn, lift your limbs as high as they will go. Curve your spine left and right as you sway your chest to each side. Think of how you might move as you swim in the warm waters off a beautiful tropical beach. If you like, reach back with one hand and hold the opposite leg, then use it to float you higher.

build up
Tiger Flow (page 32)

move forward
Three-Up Bridge Pose
(page 246)

balance out
Plough-Pose Lifts (page 208)

BLISSFUL BACKBENDS

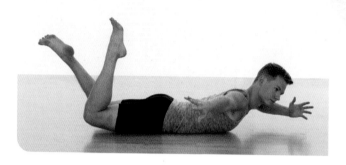

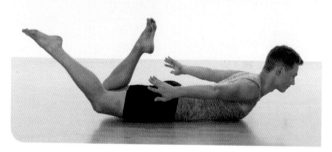

3. Continue to stretch, sway and flow organically. When your back feels warm from the healthy blood flow to all those back muscles and you are pleasantly tired, stretch back into the Child Pose (see page 288) and enjoy rounding the spine in this gentle opposite curve.

unwind
Seaweed Sway (page 106)

take care
If your back feels uncomfortable, seek further advice.
Don't practise this pose in pregnancy.

pigeon crescent pose

☆
☆
☆

This is a really enlivening pose. It's a fantastic release for one buttock, a terrific stretch for the front thigh and a backbend with a twist. Your upper and lower halves will work strongly against each other, to squeeze stagnancy out of your body and create new, vibrant, fresh good energy.

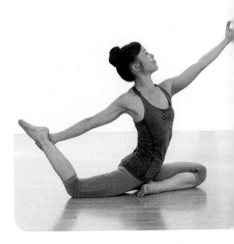

1. From all fours, bring your left knee close to your left wrist, and your left foot a little toward your right wrist. Slide your right leg back in a straight line, to come into a Pigeon Pose. It's important to be able to settle yourself toward the floor so that your hips can receive the stretch. If your left buttock doesn't touch the floor, support it with a yoga block or folded blankets. You'll need to be able to stay grounded while lifting both hands up, without tilting sideways. If your left buttock touches the floor, enhance the gluteal stretch by moving your left knee further to the left and easing your foot further forward, so that your shin is more perpendicular to your torso. Check that your right ankle is directly behind your right hip, and that your right knee is not bent out to the right. If it bends out, you need to lift your seat higher, so grab some more padding.

When you are ready, bend your right knee. Grasp your right foot with your right hand. Press your foot back against your hand and use this action to sit your torso up taller, working deeper into your backbend. Reach your left arm upward, palm up, and join the tips of your thumb and index finger. Focus now on lifting up out of the lower back and carving the concavity deeper into the mid- and upper back. Feel your breath move into the front of your torso to help it broaden, lighten and lift with each inhalation.

build up
Twisted Pigeon (page 182)

move forward
One-Legged Upward-Facing
Bow (page 248)

balance out
Seated Rotated Gate
(page 162)

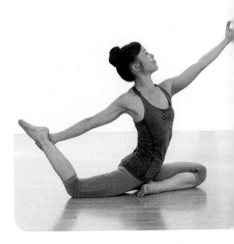

BLISSFUL BACKBENDS

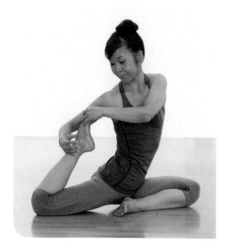

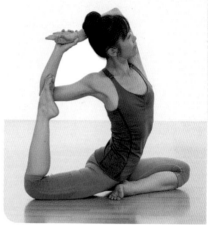

2. After five to ten breaths in the initial Pigeon Pose, move into the Pigeon Crescent Pose. Bring your right foot in close to the body. Twisting around to the right, draw your right foot in as close as possible with your left hand. Now slip your right arm behind the right ankle to nestle the foot into your elbow nook. Once you have secured the foot, reach your left arm forward, up and back, to hook the fingers of both hands together.

3. Once you are locked in, press the right side of your ribcage forward to come out of the twist as much as possible. Press your right foot back, so that you have a nice strong action to work against. Use each inhalation to bolster the squeezing-forward of your right side. At the same time, press your right foot back to develop your backbend further. Hold for five long, smooth breaths. Then come out and practise side two.

unwind
Restorative Forward Bends
(page 296)

take care
If your back feels uncomfortable, seek further advice.

camel flow

The key to a more even and lengthened-out backbend is to energize strongly upward with the chestbone when you lift, but also as you bend back. Another trick is to keep a light feeling of drawing your navel to the spine. This will lessen the compression in your lower back and bring more comfort. It will also develop the thoracic backbend, by encouraging the breath to move into the chest.

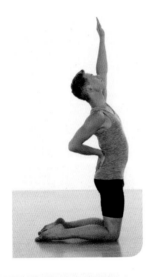

1. Kneel up, with your feet hip-width apart. Place your right palm on your sacrum (the flat, bony plate halfway between your waist and tailbone) and press lightly downward. At the same time, through this whole sequence, remember to resist back a little with the sacrum into the palm. Inhale and sweep your left arm forward and up to vertical. As you do this, lift the chest higher. Consider the lifting arm as an extension of your spine and allow its reach to lift you taller.

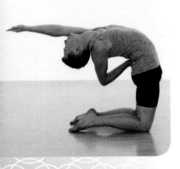

2. Keeping the ribcage lifting up out of the lower back, exhale and take your left arm back to create your backbend. Press your thigh bones forward, aiming to have them vertical. Inhale to lift your heart centre, and return your left arm to vertical. Then exhale to lower it forward and down, swapping hands so that your left palm is on your sacrum. Inhale to sweep your right arm forward and up. Exhale as you reach it back and curve into your backbend. Press your hips forward. Inhale to lift up as symmetrically as possible, then exhale to swap hands at your sacrum again. Continue for five more rounds, going a little deeper as you warm up.

build up
Salute to the Moon (page 80)

move forward
Sugar-Cane Goddess Pose
(page 120)

balance out
Heavenly Happy-Baby Pose
(page 158)

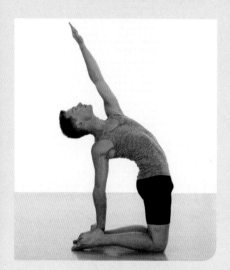
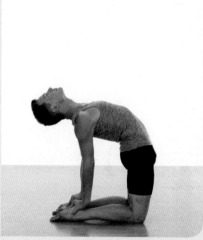

3. If you like, add a twist. Next time your left arm reaches up, look down to the right, lean back and touch your right fingertips to your left heel. Your toes can be tucked under or, for a greater challenge, un-tucked, with the tops of the feet flat on the floor. Your left arm continues to help elevate your spine. Hold for several breaths before inhaling back up, ready to change sides.

4. Try the full classic Camel Pose, by taking both hands back to your heels. Continue to lift through the centre of the chest and press the fronts of your thighs forward, while your navel moves inward. Roll your shoulders back and ensure that your neck is comfortable. Lightly drawing your chin to your throat and then looking forward and up a little works for most people.

unwind
Restorative Twist (page 292)

take care
Never work into discomfort. Don't drop your head all the way back, but maintain it in a long curve.

three-up bridge pose

Here are three ways to do a classic pose. These strong backbends are a bit like cooking pancakes: the first one out of the pan is not the best. Your first backbend might feel a little clunky, the next one gets a bit better as the body warms and opens, and by the third one things really start to feel great.

1. Sit on the floor with your knees bent up. Position your feet hip-width apart and check that the second toe of each foot points straight ahead. Roll down to lie on the floor. Walk your feet back, so that each foot sits just in front of your buttocks. Have your arms on the floor, palms down, slightly out from your hips. Lift your hips up to form your bridge shape. Tip to the right to take the weight off your left shoulder, so that you can roll it under. Then tilt to the left to roll your right shoulder under. Create a gulley of air space between your shoulder blades. Work your leg muscles to maintain the height of your hips, and move your chestbone toward your chin. Hold for five to ten long breaths. Then come down to rest. Repeat twice more or move on to step 2.

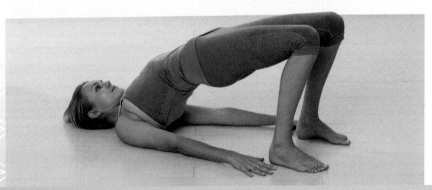

build up
Shoulder-Loving Cobra
(page 230)

move forward
One-Legged Upward-Facing
Bow (page 248)

balance out
Kinky Cobbler's Pose (page 154)

BLISSFUL BACKBENDS

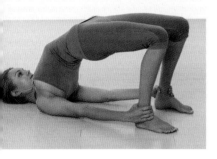 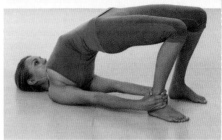

2. Bring your knees into your chest, grab the front of each ankle in each hand and replace the feet on the floor, so that they stay in, nice and close to the buttocks. Still holding onto your feet, lift your hips up once again. Once you are up, roll to each side to roll one shoulder under and then the other. Pulling against the ankles, lever your hips higher up. Reach your breastbone toward your chin. Hold for five to ten long breaths. Then come down to rest. Keeping hold of your ankles, repeat twice more or progress to step 3.

3. Lift your hips up again. Lean to the right, so that your left shoulder lifts off from the floor and, exaggerating that shoulder roll-back movement even more, reach your left hand to hold your right ankle. Then lower the left shoulder down to the floor. Using the leverage of both hands gripping, reinforce the uplift of the chest and hips. The right side of your ribcage will tend to droop, so re-double your lifting efforts here. Make your torso as symmetrical as possible. Continue to draw your shoulder blades toward each other behind your back. Keep your thigh muscles working strongly to lift your hips up. After five to ten breaths, come down again. Rest, then come up to work with both hands holding the left foot.

THREE-UP BRIDGE POSE

unwind
Cow-Pose Spirals (page 222)

take care
If your neck troubles you or is overly flattened, try folding a blanket four times, so that it is wider than your shoulders. Place it under your shoulders and upper back, so that your shoulders are lifted while your neck and head are one step lower on the floor.

one-legged upward-facing bow

This pose demands shoulder strength, which for some yogis can be their undoing; for others, it's the required flexibility that needs to develop over time. The one-legged option gives an added challenge to these two dimensions. As with all the backbends, make sure you have warmed and prepared the body with some twists, side-stretches, shoulder releases, forward bends and back-strengtheners.

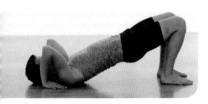

1. Lie on your back, with your knees bent and feet hip-width on the floor. Bring your palms to the floor beside your ears, fingers pointing to the shoulders. Lift your hips, directing them upward and away from your shoulders.

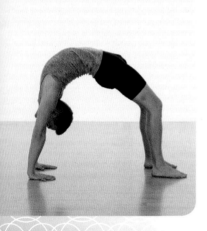

2. Catch the wave of an inhalation, press the palms into the floor and lift up. You may notice your heels lift in the air. Keeping your hips high, ease the heels down to the floor. If possible, walk them in toward your hands to make your shape more circular. Straighten your elbows as much as possible and move your chest forward, away from your buttocks. Sometimes it's easy to forget to breathe when you are upside-down, so keep your breathing steady and regular. If your toes have turned out, rearrange the feet by bringing the big toes closer together, so that the second toes can point forward. After five or more breaths, tuck your chin in and bend the elbows, to lower down with control. Rest, then repeat two more rounds. Despite the fatigue factor, each round will feel easier, as if the joints have been better lubricated.

build up
Strengthening Sun Salutation (page 76); Sage Pose with Neck Releases (page 176); Pyramid Prayer (page 140)

move forward
Drop-Backs (page 250)

balance out
Three-Step Reclining Twist (page 170)

3. On the third round, if you feel ready, lift one leg. First, turn the left foot out by 2.5cm (1in). Allow the left knee to move slightly to the left as well. Firm the left buttock, ready to bear more weight. Activate your abdominal muscles and bend your right knee as you lift your right foot off the floor. Bring your right thigh in toward your belly, keeping your knee well bent. Lengthen your right leg straight up, as vertical as your flexibility will allow. Point the toes initially, then peel your right toes back, so that the ball of the foot is the highest part of the pose. Hold for five breaths. To come out, bend the right knee in first, then lower the leg with control. Stabilize, then turn your right foot and knee out 2.5cm (1in), ready to lift the left side.

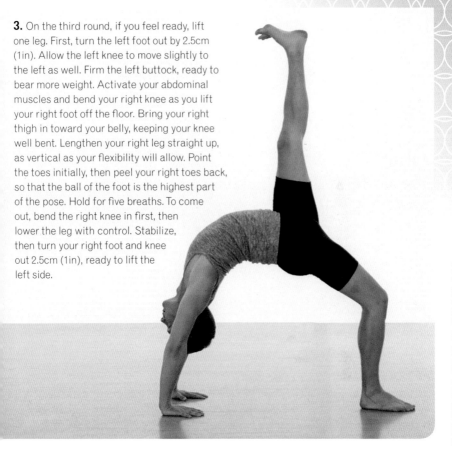

ONE-LEGGED UPWARD-FACING BOW

unwind
Yin Happy Baby (page 318)

take care
Ensure that you are well warmed up for this pose. Don't practise it during late pregnancy. Be cautious if you have high blood pressure or angina. Seek advice if you have a hiatus hernia, peptic ulcer, arthritis or any back conditions.

drop-backs

There are few poses more exhilarating than dropping back into Upward-Facing Bow. How fantastic to get there yourself, with just the help of a wall, and eventually to dispense even with that. I hope you enjoy becoming fully self-sufficient in mind and body.

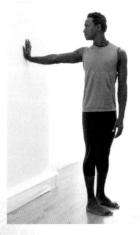

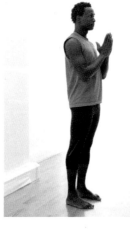

1. Stand with your back to the wall. Measure out your spacing by reaching behind to place one palm flat on the wall.

2. Turn to the front to take up your starting position. Have your feet hip-width apart, aligned so that your second toes point forward. It's really important that your thighs work well in this sequence. Switch on your front thigh muscles, so that they tighten and your kneecaps lift. Ground down well through the feet, particularly the heels. Send a message down to your heels to stay well anchored to the floor for the entire sequence.

build up	**move forward**	**balance out**
Strengthening Sun Salutation (page 76); One-Legged Upward-Facing Bow (page 248)	Pigeon Crescent Pose (page 242)	Reclining Eagle Twist (page 226)

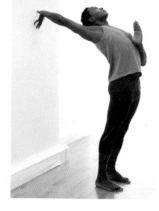

3. With your palms together at your heart, inhale and lift your chestbone up toward your thumbs. Keep this lift while you exhale. On your next inhalation reach your preferred arm up overhead and, as you exhale, take your hand back to the wall. Don't slouch into the lower back – you want to create an "up and over" feeling with the upper back, so be sure not to flatten the chest. Your legs will stay strong and straight at this point, so keep working those thighs.

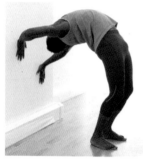

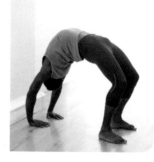

5. Once you've walked all the way down, take your palms flat to the floor into Upward-Facing Bow Pose (see page 248). Have your feet as close to the hands as possible, to make a smooth, high arch. Be as round as you can, without over-compressing the lumbar spine or needing to lift your heels. Push your palms into the floor to work the arms straight. Try to keep your feet hip-width apart and your second toes facing forward. To come out of this pose, tuck the chin in and lower yourself down to rest on your back. Repeat twice more. If you can, take both arms up and over at the same time in step 3. Work toward not needing the wall.

4. Reach up and over with your second hand, then begin to walk your hands down the wall. You will soon need to bend your knees, and you might need to walk your feet away from the wall a little.

unwind
Seated Rotated Gate (page 162). Finish with twists, lateral releases and forward bends.

take care
Warm up thoroughly first, including backbends, core-strengthening and shoulder releases. Don't practise this during pregnancy. Avoid if you have high blood pressure or angina. Seek advice if you have a hiatus hernia, peptic ulcer, arthritis or any back conditions.

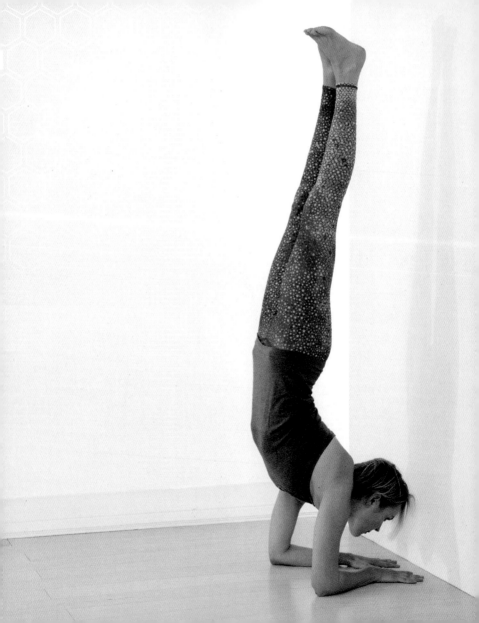

13.
UPSIDE-DOWN

It's often beneficial to look at things from a different perspective, and this is exactly what upside-down poses let us do. It's fun exploring any new yoga pose – there's something about making a new shape with your body that can shift you from being a serious adult with deadlines and commitments to a more carefree you.

It's a balancing thing, on more than just a physical level, to build the confidence and strength to fully weight-bear through the shoulders and arms. It tones muscles and builds flexibility, and you'll find that your heart pumps more. Besides building balance and core strength, yoga inversions do double-duty by giving you a work*out* plus a work-*in*.

Inversions are a boon for the digestive system, too. Our abdominal organs get suspended for that short time, and our organs of elimination seem to be given a little help. Inversions are considered to strengthen digestion by returning *agni* (the digestive fire energy) to the liver, gall-bladder and stomach – though you may want to avoid inverting if you suffer from heartburn. Inversions assist lymphatic circulation, which relies heavily on gravity and muscle movement, therefore helping the immune system. Some inversions, such as armstands and headstands, are considered "heating" to the system, giving you energy. Others, such as shoulder-stands and their follow-on poses, are considered to be cooling postures, calming for the nervous system.

Yoga folklore bills inversions as anti-ageing. While there are plenty of yoga practitioners who appear younger than their age, at the very least an inversion will send a boost of fresh oxygen and nutrient-carrying blood to your face – so I can promise you a pleasant flush.

Do read through the "cautions on inversions" overleaf. If you are in any doubt, seek help from an experienced yoga teacher. If full weight-bearing postures aren't for you right now, there are lots of achievable postures where the head is below the heart. There are many Downward-Facing Dog varieties and standing forward folds to be enjoyed.

CAUTIONS ON INVERSIONS

The headstand has been called the "father" of all postures, and the shoulder-stand the "mother". While these postures hold a historically important place in Hatha yoga practice, do remember that in the context of a modern lifestyle, these poses and their derivatives may not be appropriate for you. Modern lifestyles cause us to approach these poses from a sedentary starting point. As you have moved around upright for most of your life, weight-bearing by the head and neck needs to be built up slowly and sensibly.

Shoulder-stand- and headstand-based postures should be done when you are thoroughly warmed up, after a full-spectrum practice.

Begin with the simpler starter options shown here, and initially hold them for just a few breaths. This way your body can offer its own feedback over the next 24 hours, before you practise again. Even if you feel you have a strong, well-prepared body, be ready to leave any ego aside. It might be that certain versions of these poses don't suit you right now. It's possible to practise with good-looking form – possibly using various props and alignment tweaks – yet still notice that these poses don't suit you perfectly. In this case, work with an experienced teacher.

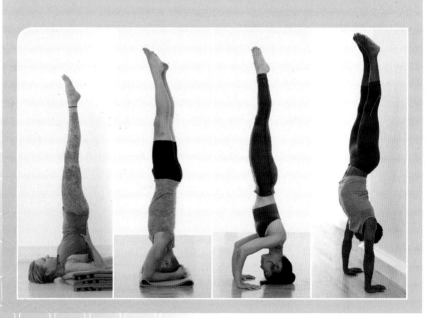

TO INVERT OR NOT TO INVERT?

Avoid inversions if you have degenerative conditions of the upper body, any concerns about current or previous neck injuries or pains, shoulder aches, weakness, excess tightness or imbalance. Seek advice first from a professional in cases of a slipped (herniated) disc or any inflammation of the back. Avoid upside-down postures if you have a severe heart condition, high blood pressure, glaucoma, a detached retina, inner-ear discharge or severe sinus infection. Don't practise while you have a headache. Seek further advice if you have osteoporosis: you could develop a strategy around inversions with an experienced teacher.

It's not recommended to invert during menstruation. Going against the natural direction of flow can slow down the body's process of elimination. During pregnancy, it's possible to practise headstands and shoulder-stands during the first and second trimesters (but never after 35 weeks), as long as you have had regular practice of them to date. However, many pregnant women find the desire to invert drops away during pregnancy, so feel free to give these dramatic-looking poses a miss for the duration. If you do want to continue during pregnancy, you need to be able to lift up your legs with graceful control, without jolting at all. For the headstand and tripod balances, stay at the wall, so that there is no risk of you toppling over.

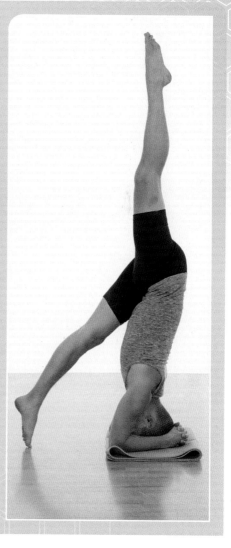

☆ starter shoulder-stand

This is a great way to get to know Shoulder-Stand safely. It suits beginners and those carrying extra weight or with weak abdominal muscles. As you come up in such a controlled way, this method can also suit pregnant women up to 35 weeks.

1. Fold three large blankets to 80 x 50cm (30 x 20in) and about 10cm (4in) thick. Place your blanket stack with the wide side parallel to the wall. It should be about 25cm (10in) from the wall, or a little further away if you are very tall. To come into position, sit side-on to the wall, with your left hip and shoulder touching it. One buttock will be on the blankets and the other hovering above the floor. Lean back on both hands and swivel on your seat as you lift your legs up the wall.

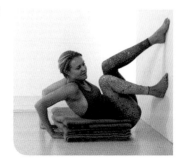

2. Lie yourself back, to bring your legs together up the wall. Now double-check your position on the blanket. It's not necessary to have your buttocks touching the wall. What is important is that your head is on the lower level and your shoulders are on the upper level. Ensure that your shoulders are 5cm (2in) from the edge of the blanket. Roll to the side to come out, if necessary, and tweak the blanket distance. Once you have it right, look down the front of your body to check that your heels, pubic bone and throat centre are all in one line. This posture, with or without the blanket, is called *Viparita Karani*. It's a little bit magical, with its restorative effects, and some days it's enough to rest here for ten to 20 minutes.

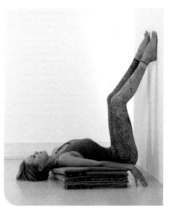

UPSIDE-DOWN

build up	**move forward**	**balance out**
Seated Neck Stretch and Strengthen (page 134)	Basic Shoulder-Stand (page 258)	Kinky Cobbler's Pose (page 154)

3. To continue to your Starter Shoulder-Stand, slide your feet down the wall and bend your knees to about 90 degrees. Press your feet to the wall to lift your hips up. Proceed carefully and check how your neck is feeling. It's important that it doesn't feel stretched taut, and it should always feel comfortable. Take your palms to your lower back.

4. Walk your feet up the wall to straighten your legs. Bearing more weight through your wrists, detach one foot from the wall, then the other, to reach your legs straight up. Congratulations: you are in Shoulder-Stand.

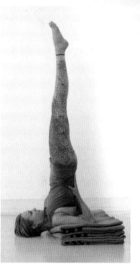

5. Continually check that your neck is still feeling comfortable. If you feel that your neck is too flexed for comfort with your legs more to the vertical, fold at your hips to bring your feet forward and your hips back. Start by holding for half a minute, then build up with repeated regular practice over the weeks and months to a five-minute hold.

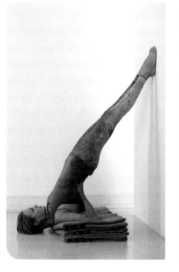

unwind
Restorative Twist (page 292)

take care
Shoulder-Stands are best not practised during menstruation or in pregnancy beyond 35 weeks. Seek personalized advice if you have any neck or shoulder issues. See page 254 for the cautions on inversions.

STARTER SHOULDER-STAND

basic shoulder-stand

Using the blankets in Starter Shoulder-Stand (see page 256) helps to ensure that your neck isn't pushed too far into flexion while weight-bearing. Over weeks and month of practice you will be able to remove the blankets, one by one. The time to forgo them is once you have a sustained, regular Shoulder-Stand practice, where your neck feels good during and afterward.

1. Position yourself on the blanket stack so that your shoulders are about 8cm (3in) away from the edges, with your head on the lower level. Bend your knees and place your hands, palms down, beside your hips. Press down on your palms and contract your abdominal muscles to lift your legs and hips up in the air. Keeping your knees bent, continue to roll up the spine until your knees hover above your head. Bring your hands to your sacrum. Keep looking straight up. Acclimatize here for several breaths. Check that your neck is feeling fine. If so, proceed; if not, come out.

2. Without turning your head to the side, tilt a little to your right to slightly release the left shoulder. Roll it back, so that you get a good shoulder tuck-under on that left side. Now weight-bear more through the left, so that you can roll the right shoulder under, then return to symmetry. The idea is to create a gulley between your shoulder blades and

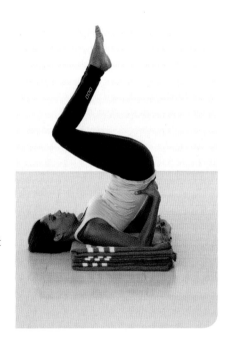

UPSIDE-DOWN

build up	**move forward**	**balance out**
Starter Shoulder-Stand (page 256)	Plough-Pose Lifts (page 208)	Neck Releases after Inversions (page 262)

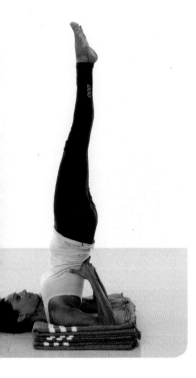

bring your elbows closer together, which will allow your torso to lift up more. Eventually your upper-arm bones will be parallel and your hands will be able to walk down from your sacrum to hold your mid-back.

3. A bend at the hips with the legs at an angle and plenty of weight in your hands is safest, while your body gets accustomed to regular Shoulder-Stand practice. Once you have set up your foundation and are feeling comfortable, you will be ready to lift your legs higher and will find the angles that suit your body best. Move the chest to your chin, lift more through the front of the torso and elevate the legs, so that the whole shape is more vertical. Whatever your shape, remember that you are getting all the great benefits of Shoulder-Stand, so leave the ego out of it and choose whichever option truly suits your body best. Start with holding for 30 seconds, then build up to five minutes with regular practice. Over those five minutes you will need to make small adjustments to maintain your lift and symmetry. Certainly do this, but try not to fidget unnecessarily. Focus on lifting through long, straight legs, on your breath and on your stillness. Then come out and practise the Shoulder-Stand counterposes (see page 262, Neck Releases After Inversions).

unwind
Head-Beyond-the-Knee Pose
(page 160)

take care
Shoulder-Stands are best not practised during menstruation or in pregnancy beyond 35 weeks. Seek personalized advice if you have any neck or shoulder issues. See page 254 for the cautions on inversions.

plough, half-lotus plough and spider pose

There are so many interesting options when you progress on from Shoulder-Stand.
Here are a few to follow on with.

plough pose

From Shoulder-Stand, fold at the hips
and lower your legs overhead. If you are
flexible in your forward bending, you may
be able to touch your feet to the floor,
toes tucked under. If you can't touch
down, continue to support your back with
your palms. In this case, allow your knees
to bend while the toes float. You can allow
the spine to round softly in this hovering
position, which is more restful. However,
if you can touch your toes down, lift more
through the spine to bring it a little more
vertical, so that the hips stack more over
the shoulders. Then interlace your fingers
and reach your arms back along the floor.
Your arms and shoulder line will create
a tripod of support, making a base from
which to lift the torso. This pose works
using your three blankets initially; then
with time and experience, and if it suits
your neck, you can reduce to none.

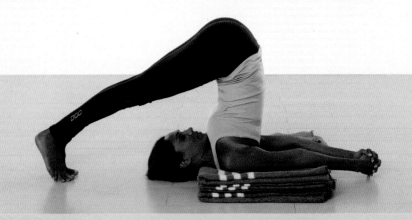

build up
Basic Shoulder-Stand
(page 258)

move forward
Basic Headstand (page 268)

balance out
Neck Releases after Inversions
(page 262)

UPSIDE-DOWN

half-lotus plough

From Shoulder-Stand, with the legs fairly
vertical, rotate the left thigh bone externally
to turn your left leg out. Then bend the left
knee and bring your foot to the front of
your right thigh. Use one hand to maintain
your lower back support, while you bring
the other hand up to help nestle your left
heel into the right groin, or as close as
possible on the upper thigh. Once your foot
is in place, lower your right leg overhead,
possibly bringing your right toes to the floor.
Check there are no messages of discomfort
coming from your left knee as you do this.
Extend the arms away along the floor and
interlace your fingers. Hold for up to one
minute, before returning to Shoulder-Stand
to practise the second side.

spider pose

This increases the forward bend and
is only suitable if you are comfortable
in Plough Pose without blankets.
Take the Plough Pose with your
toes touched down and your hands
supporting your back. Walk both feet
to the left. Check that your neck is
feeling comfortable. Slowly lower your
knees to the floor, just beside your
left ear, and rest the tops of your feet
on the floor. Reach your arms away
along to floor. Interlace your fingers
and press your arms down, to allow
more lift through your torso. Hold for
five to ten breaths, then move into the
second side.

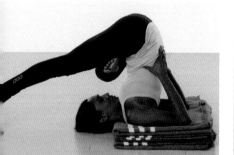

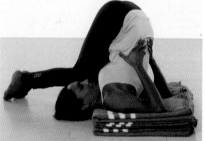

unwind
Three-Step Reclining Twist
(page 170)

take care
Shoulder-Stand variations are best not practised during
menstruation or in pregnancy beyond 35 weeks. Seek
personalized advice, if you have any neck or shoulder issues.
See page 254 for the cautions on inversions.

☆ neck releases after inversions

This sequence is really valuable. It helps keep your neck safe and happy after practising the strong flexion that occurs in Shoulder-Stand and the Plough Pose, and after the weight-bearing that occurs during Headstand and its variations.

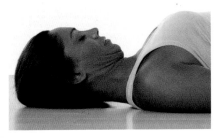

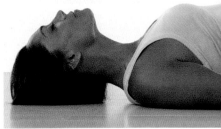

1. Once you have come out of your inversion, lie flat on your back with your knees bent up. If you are using blankets, move down so that your head and back are on the same level. Come into position without twisting your neck to either side, as it's important to first release the neck in a forward and backward direction. Press your chin in toward your throat to flatten your neck toward the floor. Feel how the head slides away from the shoulders to allow the neck to lengthen. Stay for two breaths.

2. Next arch your neck vertebrae and slide the base of your skull toward your shoulders slightly. Hold for two breaths. Then repeat the neck flexion and extension movements several more times each.

3. Fish Pose is great to do after Shoulder-Stand. Lengthen your legs out straight. Slide one hand under each buttock, palms down. Drawing the chin toward the throat, lift up through the chest and come up to rest on your forearms. You will be looking forward at this stage. Then take your torso back as you lift your chin and let the crown of the head move toward the floor. As the angle of your elbows increases, the crown of your head may lightly touch the floor. Ensure that most of the weight is borne by the forearms and lower body. Hold for five to ten breaths. To come out, lift the head just enough to un-wedge it from the floor, and lower yourself all the way down, to lie on your back. Hug your knees into your belly and practise another couple of neck flexions (step 1) and extensions (step 2).

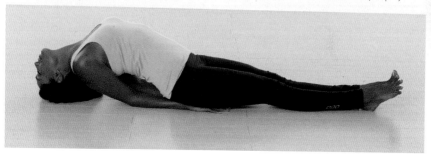

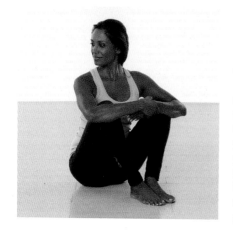

4. After your neck releases, roll your whole body to the side, head included. You still have not twisted the neck. Come up to sitting. Once you are sitting, you can turn your head from side to side. Head-Beyond-the-Knee Pose (see page 160) is one of my favourite postures to practise after inversions.

☆ starter headstand

This pose, also called the Hare Pose, is great, as it's fairly easy to limit the amount of weight the head bears. The neck vertebrae get to practise weight-bearing, as insurance against osteoporosis later in life. It's also superb preparation for Headstand, as you practise the correct lifting action at the shoulders.

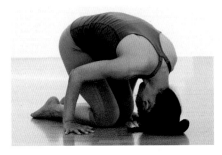 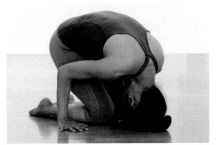

1. Kneel and fold your torso forward into the Child Pose (see page 288). Bring your hands to the floor, shoulder-width apart, positioned with your fingers roughly on the same line as the forehead. Lift your hips up as you roll from your forehead to the crown of your head. Try to rest on the anterior fontanelle – where the soft part at the top of a baby's head is. Aim to have the bones of your neck fairly vertical. If they are not, roll back down to your forehead, then adjust by moving your forehead in closer to your knees before coming back into the pose.

2. Now practise the correct setting of the shoulders. Slide your shoulder blades toward your waist and lift the tops of your shoulders away from the ears, so that they form a horizontal line. Have your upper-arm bones parallel, so that your elbows point straight backward. This will let you better control how much weight is on your head. Aim for it to take around 20 per cent of the weight, but test the waters by doing less. Lift your back to a high, rounded shape. After three to ten breaths, rest back down to Child Pose or, if it feels right, proceed to the next stage.

build up	move forward	balance out
Seated Neck Stretch and Strengthen (page 134)	Basic Headstand (page 268)	Neck Releases after Inversions (page 262), steps 1 and 2

UPSIDE-DOWN

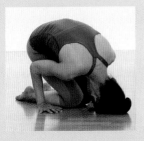 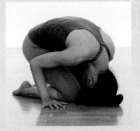 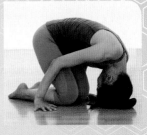

3. Still pressing the palms to the floor and lifting the shoulders up and away, roll down toward your forehead an inch or so. Then start to circle around the crown of your head. Let your hips move sideways, back and around, as you create slow circles. Enjoy this nice head massage. After several loops, circle back the other way. After three more rounds, roll down to Child Pose or, if you are ready, move on to the full posture.

4. With the weight once again through the crown of your head, interlace your hands behind your back. Lift your arms to vertical or beyond, and use this reach to lessen the pressure on the head a little. Stay for ten breaths, then reposition the palms on the floor to help you roll down and rest in Child Pose for a minute. When you are ready to sit up, roll up through the spine so that the head comes into position last of all.

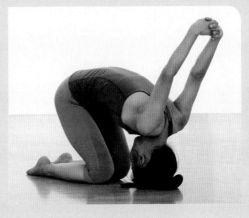

unwind
Restorative Twist (page 292)

take care
See page 254 for the cautions on inversions.

headless headstand

This ingenious practice has many elements and benefits of the full Headstand, but without any weight-bearing on the head. It lets you get used to going upside-down and regulating your breathing while you are there. Many people love it, but for the first few times stay for only a few breaths, to be sure it suits your shoulders.

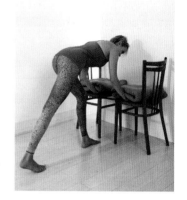

1. Take two strong identical chairs and position them by a wall, facing each other. The seat edges should be about 16cm (6in) apart, just enough for you to slip your head through, but narrow enough to support your shoulders. Fold two matching blankets so that they create a broad pad about 10cm (4in) high. Ensure they are exactly the same height, as they will become your base. Slide your hands in under the pads, so that the palms are resting on the seat of the chair. Your wrists will be near the front of the chair.

2. Your chairs should be just wide enough apart for you to slip your head in between them. Do this now, and position your shoulders about halfway along the chair edge (deeper in than your wrists). Step your feet away and let the whole top of your shoulder line rest on the padded supports. Lift up to tiptoes and walk your feet in toward the chairs. At a certain point you won't be able to walk in anymore without bending your knees. This is the place to kick up from. Lift one leg up as high as possible.

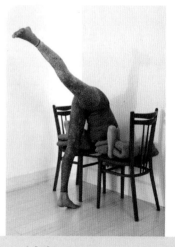

build up	move forward	balance out
Starter Handstand (page 264)	Basic Headstand (page 268)	Seated Rotated Gate (page 162)

3. Bend the other knee and, when you are ready, kick up that leg and then the other (or, with experience, lightly float your legs up). Take both heels to the wall. In time you can practise not touching the wall at all. Once you are up, get as symmetrical as possible. It helps to have someone stand back opposite you, to check your alignment. Keep your breathing long and steady. Often the reason people come out of inversions is not that they were physically unable to hold it for longer, but because they forgot to keep breathing. Practise moving your feet away from the wall, to free-balance. Stay for three breaths initially, building up to a minute over repeated regular practice.

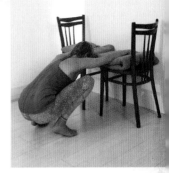

4. To come down, scissor one leg forward, toes tucked under, and land lightly down. Once both feet are on the floor, step backward, releasing the head from the chairs. Take a low squat or kneeling position for a minute, until you are ready to come up.

unwind
Restorative Forward Bends
(page 296)

take care
See page 254 for the cautions on inversions.

HEADLESS HEADSTAND

basic headstand

Known as the king of the yoga postures, Headstand is considered to be calming to the nervous system, although it can also bring a fresh zing to your day. Do read the "take care" cautions below, to see if it will suit you. Start off using a wall and, once you feel practised enough, move to the centre of the room.

1. Fold a yoga mat to form a large rectangle. Place it between you and the wall, then kneel in front of it. Position your elbows on it shoulder-width apart and interlace your fingers, about 20 cm (8 inches) from the wall. Check that your wrists are vertical, with the thin edge facing up. Press the underside of the wrist into the floor, so there is no rolling in or out of the wrists. Place the back of your head into the arch created by your hands. Ensure it's the crown of the head that touches the floor, not the forehead.

While still kneeling, practise lifting your shoulders away from the floor. Press down evenly through the forearms, creating a triangle of support, while the shoulders lift up and away to encourage minimal compression of the neck. When you can do this action, you are ready to lift your hips and straighten your legs. If you lift your hips and find that you can't help your shoulders collapsing down, or your neck comes out of its natural curve, then stop for now, until you build up your flexibility and strength.

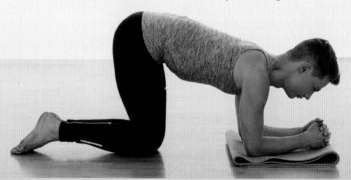

build up
Warm up with a balanced practice first, including Seated Neck Stretch and Strengthen (page 134), Starter Headstand (page 264) or Headless Headstand (page 266).

move forward
Tripod to One-Legged Crow Pose (page 278)

balance out
Neck Releases after Inversions (page 262), steps 1 and 2

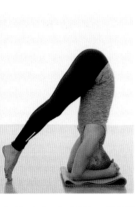

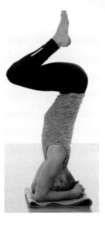

2. On tiptoes, walk your feet in until you can't go further. This is the point where you feel the readiness to lift. Your shoulders and hips will be lined up above your ears. Continue to press the forearms down and the shoulders up. Firm your abdominal muscles.

3. Bend your knees to allow your feet to float up. Bring your knees in toward your abdomen. Aim for the arms to take 70 per cent of the weight and the head just 30 per cent. Stabilize here.

4. If you feel steady, come all the way up. "Unfold" your legs by first pointing your knees upward, so that your heels are near your buttocks.

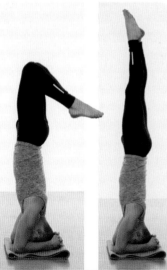

5. Now straighten your legs in the air. Start with a 30-second hold. Before you build up to longer holds, seek advice from a qualified teacher who can check your alignment. Once you are up, ensure your hips stay symmetrical. Keep your shoulders working away from the ears, to limit the weight on the head, and press the floor away with your arms. Extend through the feet, to keep the sense of lift. When you are strong here you will feel lighter. To come down, reverse the steps you took to get up: fold at the knees, then hinge at the hips to bring your toes to the floor lightly and with control. Rest in the Child Pose (see page 288) for a full minute.

BASIC HEADSTAND

unwind

Legs-up-the-Wall Pose (page 298)

take care

Avoid Headstand if you have concerns about current or previous neck injuries, pains, headaches, shoulder aches or excess tightness. Avoid inversions if you have eye issues such as a detached retina or a risk of glaucoma. Extra care must be taken during pregnancy, so make sure to work with an experienced teacher.

headstand variations

Once you have mastered Headstand and can do it with ease away from the wall, jazz up your practice with these options.

headstand split twist

From a stable Basic Headstand (see page 268), scissor your legs so that your right leg goes forward and the left goes back. As you do this, each hip will move toward its leg, coming a little out of its starting point of horizontal alignment. Ensure the back leg remains straight, and do your best to ease it down as low as your front leg. Now move into the twist by sending the right leg to the left. Once you have twisted, return your attention to your legs. Internally rotate both thighs. Then energize both legs away from each other, by reaching out through the balls of the feet while fanning the toes back toward the midline. Hold for up to a minute, before lifting back up to Headstand, ready for the second side.

build up
Do a full warming practice with Seated Neck Stretch and Strengthen (page 134), a selection of abdominal strengthening practices and Basic Headstand (page 268)

move forward
Forearm Balance (page 276)

balance out
Child Pose (page 288)

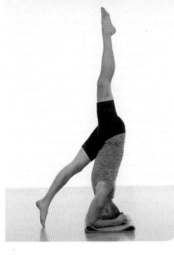

one-legged headstand split

From a steady Basic Headstand position, extend upward through the right leg. Rotate the left leg outward, so that the toes point to the left. Lower the left leg out to the side, possibly as far as touching the toes to the floor and pressing the left heel away. Continue to lift the shoulder line away from the floor. Lighten the amount of weight on the head by keeping an even pressure through left and right forearms and pressing down. Maintain the internal thigh rotation of the right leg, reaching it up and away. After five to ten breaths, lift your left leg, stabilize, then practise side two.

headstand crunches

This variation will really wake up the abdominal muscles. From your Basic Headstand, exhale to lower both straight legs and hover the feet just above the floor. You are using your legs as resistance for your abdominal muscles to work against. As you do this, your hips will move backward from their

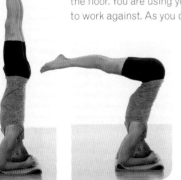

starting alignment over the shoulders. Inhale as you hold the legs low, then exhale and lift them to vertical. Inhale once you are upright, then exhale to lower again. The slower you go, the more strengthening this is, as you are not relying on momentum or gravity. Repeat for up to ten rounds, paying attention to the strength in your shoulders and maintaining their lift. Remember: in Headstand most of the weight should be on the forearms and hand edges, not on the head itself.

unwind
Neck Releases after Inversions (page 262); Corkscrew Twist (page 172)

take care
See page 254 for the cautions on inversions.

☆
☆
starter handstand

This preparation for Handstand is a safe and controlled way to find out if you are ready for the next stage of kicking up. Although it's easier in some ways, you may find forming the table-like shape against the wall requires even more strength in the core and shoulders than the next stage! Try it out, and enjoy turning your world upside-down.

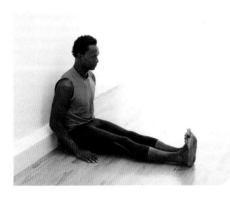 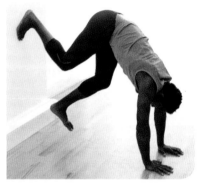

1. To measure out your spacing, sit with your back to a wall and check where your heels come to. Then come to all fours and place the heels of your hands at the point where your heels were. Position your hands shoulder-width apart, with the fingers spread wide. Press down evenly through the knuckles of all the fingers. Once the knuckles are anchored, exaggerate the pressing of the pads of the fingers into the floor. These actions will help to keep your wrists safe.

2. Tuck your toes under and lift your knees, so that you are in an inverted V-shape. It will feel like a shortened Classic Downward-Facing Dog Pose (see page 58), with your hands a little closer to the feet than usual. With both knees up, take one foot to the wall. While you press the foot into the wall, lift your second foot to the wall and walk it up a little higher than the first.

build up	**move forward**	**balance out**
Dog to Plank Flow (page 210)	Handstand at the Wall (page 274)	Seated Rotated Gate (page 162)

UPSIDE-DOWN

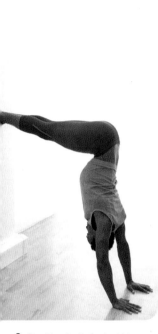

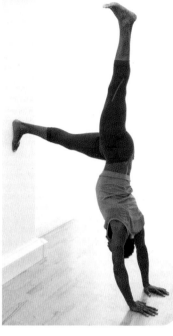

4. Get more of the upside-down feeling by taking one leg up to vertical. Reach up through that leg to press the sole of the foot as high as possible. Remember your breath – often, it's running out of air that will make you come down early. Build up your time in Starter Handstand to up to a minute. Once you are done, walk your legs down the wall to bring your feet to the floor again. Bend the knees and come to rest in Child Pose (see page 288), arms by your side. Then sit up and circle your wrists in both directions.

3. Position both feet at hip height, so that your legs are parallel. Press the floor away with your palms. Keep your abdominal muscles engaged, to help you hold this steady. It is actually easier to walk your feet higher up, so you can take that option while you build strength.

unwind
Resting Cobbler's Poses
(page 284)

take care
Seek advice if you suffer from wrist strain or weakness.

handstand at the wall

This might be something you haven't done since you were a kid in the playground – it's fun and enlivening. It can remind us all of the curious, light-hearted, childlike spirit that we carry with us always. Let it remind you that this spirit can triumph over those day-to-day tasks that grown-ups need to do.

1. Kneel in front of a wall and position your hands shoulder-width apart, so that your fingertips are about 15cm (6in) from the wall. Spread your fingers wide, and even out the pressure between the inner and outer palms by pressing your thumb side down a little more. Tuck your toes under and lift your knees, so that you come to a Classic Downward-Facing Dog Pose (see page 58). Walk your feet in toward your hands. Bring your shoulders above your knuckles and lift your hips as high as you can.

Lift one leg in the air as high as possible. If you feel you can maintain the strength and the lift in the shoulders, you are ready to kick up. If you feel you might collapse, then this is far enough for today. Instead, continue practising Downward-Facing Dog, the Plank position (see page 77) and general shoulder-stretching poses, to get ready over time.

build up
Plough-Pose Lifts (page 208)

move forward
Forearm Balance (page 276)

balance out
Yin Child with a Twist (page 315)

UPSIDE-DOWN

274

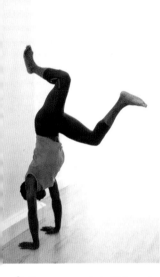
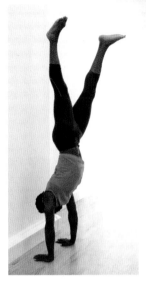
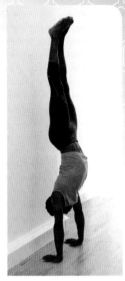

2. If you are ready to kick up, bend both knees. Contract your abdominal muscles to prepare to lift, as they will help the journey skyward. Use the lower leg to give a strong, confident kick, so that you can float both legs up as you straighten them. Once the top leg touches the wall, your second leg will follow on and both heels will touch the wall. Keep your abdominal muscles activated,

so that over time you can bring one leg – and then both – away from the wall to free-balance. Hold for up to a minute, then scissor your legs to come down. Bend your knees to the floor and take your hips to your heels, to rest in Child Pose (see page 288). When you sit up, circle your wrists in both directions to release any strain.

unwind
Resting Pigeon (page 294)

take care
Seek advice if you suffer from wrist strain or weakness.

HANDSTAND AT THE WALL

forearm balance

This pose feels like such a delight when all the elements combine well. When the shoulders are strong enough to support you confidently, yet flexible enough to allow a flight-like lift, you can soar upward with joy and lightness. I love to practise a set of abdominal-strengtheners before this pose, as they help enormously in free-balancing.

1. Kneel in front of a wall and bring your elbows to the floor, no wider than your shoulders. Have your index finger pointing forward, about 10cm (4in) from the wall. Adjust your forearms so that they are parallel, then spread the fingers and root down, particularly through the inner wrists and thumb knuckles. This will prevent the thumbs from sliding toward each other, which tends to happen here.

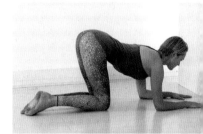

2. Tuck the toes under and lift the knees to come into an inverted V-shape. On tiptoes, and with the knees bent, lift up from the shoulders, so that the crown of the head passively lifts away from the floor. As your shoulder muscles work, develop your shoulder flexibility by moving your armpits in and up toward the fronts of your thighs. Aim to create a straight line from your elbows through your shoulders to your hips. If your head is on the floor, you need to develop your flexibility (with Pyramid Prayer, see page 140) and your strength (with Three-Legged Dogs, see page 62) before progressing to step 3.

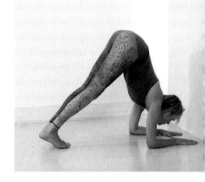

build up
Seated Yogic Roll-Downs (page 204); Pyramid Prayer (page 140); Three-Legged Dog (page 62)

move forward
One-Legged Upward-Facing Bow (page 248)

balance out
Reclining Eagle Twist (page 226)

3. Walk your feet toward your elbows a little. Then realign again, by lifting the shoulders away from the floor to create that clean line from the elbow through the shoulder to the hip. Walk in again until you can't walk any more. This is your natural kicking point. Lift one leg up. Bend both knees, then kick up while you straighten both knees. A strong, committed kick up will take both legs together to the wall. At no time during Forearm Balance will your head touch down on the floor – that's a sign to work on your flexibility some more. Each time you practise, keep your body in balance by changing your kicking leg.

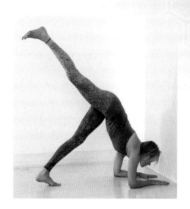
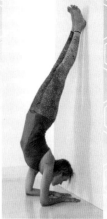

4. The next step is to move one foot, then both feet, away from the wall to a free-balance. Once you are able to hold the full balance for one minute, you can move 40cm (15in) away from the wall and practise kicking up to the free-balance. When you do this, the leading leg will momentarily come close to touching the wall, only to be immediately counterbalanced by the trailing leg. Draw both legs together, contract your core muscles and press the balls of the feet up to the sky, to contribute to the lift that your shoulders are continually giving. Continue to press the floor away actively with the forearms, inner wrists and fingertips. Stay for up to 20 slow breaths, then scissor the legs to come down lightly, with toes tucked under. Rest in the Child Pose (see page 288).

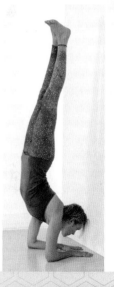

FOREARM BALANCE

unwind
Yin Shoulder Stretches
(page 322)

take care
Seek advice before practising this if you have shoulder pain. This pose demands both strength and flexibility, so be prepared to work on whichever of these elements is missing for you.

tripod to one-legged crow pose

This highly complex sequence requires focus, strength, spatial awareness and confidence. Be sure to build up appropriately first. Become proficient in the Crow Pose (see page 146) and, for the inversion element, the Basic Headstand (see page 268), before you attempt the Tripod Pose.

1. Come into the Tripod Pose from hands and knees, with palms on the floor shoulder-width apart. If you are not planning to drop into the Crow Pose, you might practise just in front of a wall. Take the crown of your head to the floor. It's essential to pressurize your palms into the floor and lift your shoulders up and away from it. This will provide better support for the neck and reduce the weight-bearing load on the head. Keep your arm bones parallel to ensure your elbows don't splay apart. With toes tucked under, lift your knees in the air and, with straight legs, walk forward on tiptoes as far as you can, with the hips remaining high. Now bring one knee to your upper arm, then do the same on the second side.

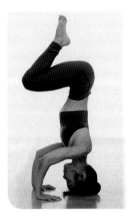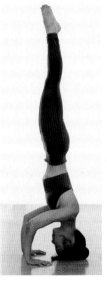

2. You are now ready to squeeze your knees together, inhale and, powering on your abdominal muscles, bring both legs straight up in the air. Congratulations: you are now in your Tripod Pose, so breathe and enjoy balancing there. Continue to lift your shoulders away from your ears, and press down actively on the palms to lessen the load through your head and neck.

UPSIDE-DOWN

build up
Seated Yogic Roll-Downs (page 204); Crow Pose (page 146); Basic Headstand (page 268)

move forward
Forearm Balance (page 276)

balance out
Neck Releases after Inversions (page 262)

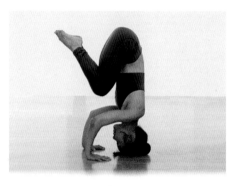

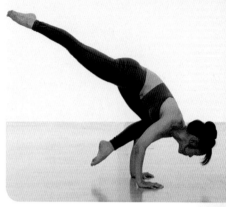

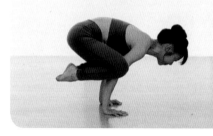

3. Come into the Crow Pose. With your abdominal muscles on, bend your knees to bring your heels toward your buttocks. Then, moving the front ribcage into the body, fold at the hips to bring your knees toward your torso. Next, lower your knees to wrap them around your upper arms. Keep your toes lifted as you lower your hips. Bring your chest forward, to lift your head off the ground in Crow Pose.

4. Preparing to come into your One-Legged Crow, seek to straighten your arms as much as possible. Squeeze your arms toward each other and lift your hips higher in the air. Draw up with your abdominal muscles. Actively reach your right leg back and establish a counterbalance with the chest, to shift your weight forward. Bring your extended knee back to the arm, and practise the second side. If this is too challenging, start instead with both sets of toes lightly on the floor and then extend a single leg away in turn. This will give you a great sense of where you need to stabilize, in order to be able to hold the full arm balance.

unwind
Revolved Happy Pose
(page 174)

take care
Warm up thoroughly with a well-rounded yoga practice first. Avoid the Tripod Pose if you have a shoulder or neck weakness, injury or imbalance. Seek advice before practising if you have any neck, wrist or shoulder issues.

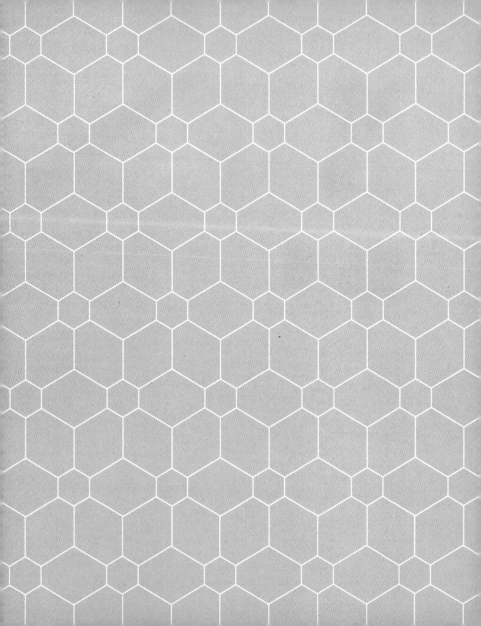

Part 3

YOGA ENERGY: YIN – THE QUIET PRACTICES

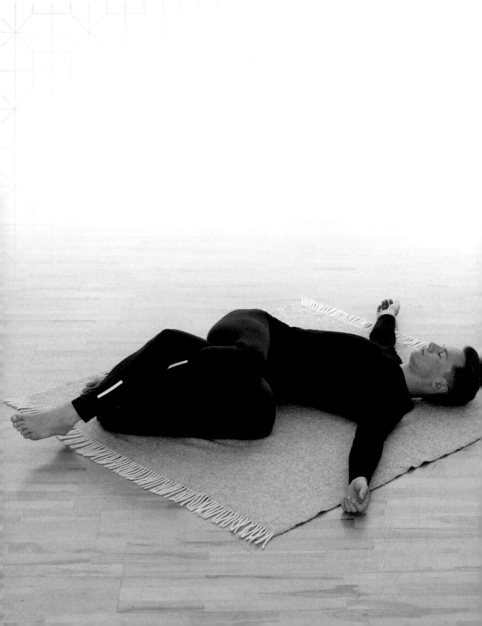

RESTORATIVE YOGA

Restorative yoga is a category of poses where you position your body in supported postures and then relax into them for two to 20 minutes. You should feel no pain and there should be minimal intensity. Your body is allowed to open gently. Some parts of your body get to expand, while others get to condense. You de-stress, because your "rest and restore" nervous system can switch on, and your "fight or flight" stress-based nervous system can clock out for the duration.

It sounds easy – too easy perhaps. And physically it is pretty easy. Sometimes the real challenge lies in just letting go of the thinking, and some people find this a little confrontational, as the mind keeps ticking over. For this reason I have given you a job to do on each page: "what to do while you're there". It's to keep the mind busy with something wholesome, so that the rest of you get on with the job of relaxing.

Ultimately, your body will sleep and your mind will simply watch.

If you have a chronic or recent injury, do seek guidance before practising yoga poses. Otherwise, who does restorative yoga suit? It suits those who are exhausted, tired, have trouble sleeping or difficulty in letting go of control. It suits many people who have a chronic disease, are under stress or may experience stress in the future. It suits teenagers, university students, parents, people who work, those who overwork and those who don't work. It suits grown-ups, whether you feel young, old or very old. Are you getting my message? It suits just about anyone who lives in the modern world.

Try out a complete practice once a week, following these poses in the order in which they are presented. Or book-end your active practice with a couple of these poses each time.

☆ resting cobbler's poses

Enjoy one of these restful postures while you centre yourself at the start of your yoga practice.

cobbler's pose over two crossed bolsters

This softly supported hip-opening pose is delightful when you need to re-centre.

1. Take two yoga bolsters or fold two blankets to form a wedge about 80 x 30 x 15cm (30 x 12 x 6in). Cross the two props to make a T-shape, with the crossways bolster underneath. The top bolster will be on an incline, to support your spine and form a pillow for your head.

2. Roll up a blanket to form a roll about 1.2m (4ft) long. Sit so that your lower back is touching the end of the top bolster, and place the soles of your feet together so that your knees bend out wide. Lift the knees and wrap the blanket over your feet and tuck it in under your ankles. Snake it up to your outer hips, so they are supported when you drop your knees away from each other.

3. Lay your spine back on the top bolster. Your buttocks will be on the floor; ensure that your sacrum is well supported by the bolster. Your head will be higher than your heart, which in turn will be higher than your hips. Lay your arms out to the sides, palms up and fingers softly curled. If you are not perfectly comfortable, make adjustments as required. Cover your eyes with an eye-pillow or light cloth. Stay for five to ten minutes. To come out of the pose, use your hand to help bring one thigh up and slowly roll out to the side.

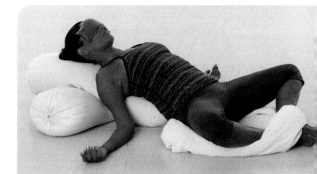

what to do while you're there

To count yourself into a relaxed state: breathe in for a count of four beats, then exhale for four beats. Do this for five or ten rounds, counting with your thumb against your fingers, if you like. Then increase the timing to breathe in for five and exhale for five. After your five or ten rounds, when it feels right, increase your counts to six. Continue lengthening both inhalations and exhalations, through seven until you reach eight,

bound cobbler's pose

The belt gives a lovely traction to the lower back and allows deeper work into the hips.

1. Sit with your back to a bolster, or blankets folded to form a pad about 80 x 30 x 15cm (30 x 12 x 6in). Guide a soft yoga belt around your lower back, above both inner thighs, over the ankles and under the feet. Tie it up beside one ankle, so that the free end of the belt extends toward your hips.

2. Leave the belt fairly loose as you lie back on the bolster. If you need a pillow, use an extra folded blanket to support the head and neck. Now tighten the belt by pulling on the band. Make sure it provides even support around both hips, thighs and ankles. Rest your arms out to the side and check that you feel warm, supported and able to let your body go heavy and relaxed. Stay for five to ten minutes.

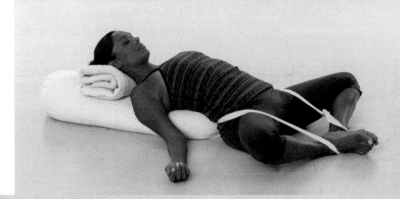

where you will have slowed your breathing rate by half. Reduce the count if it feels at all stressful or like hard work – remember: the aim is to de-stress the system, not add more stress in.

take care

Don't stay in the pose if feels uncomfortable. Activate your stretched muscles before you move to come out of the pose.

RESTING COBBLER'S POSES

☆ blissful banana

This is one of my all-time favourite postures. It stretches the side body, re-sets the breathing and restores the mind – and all without any effort. I hope you enjoy it as much as I do.

1. Fold up a blanket to form your pillow. It needs to be as high as the distance from your shoulder tip to your ear – around 7–18cm (3–7in). Take a yoga bolster or fold up a blanket to form a pad about 80 x 30 x 15cm (30 x 12 x 6in). Lay your left side over it, so that your buttock comfortably touches the floor. Allow a gap of about 15cm (6in) for your left shoulder to snuggle into, then place your pillow under your head. Extend your left arm out in front, palm up. Check that you haven't pinned the left shoulder back and under. To relieve any squashing, reach the armpit forward a little. Bring a soft bend into your knees, so that you don't have to worry about balancing. Take your right arm up and over in line with your ear, to bring your palm to a yoga brick or two offering a support 8–15cm (3–6in) in height. Adjust for comfort and rest here for two minutes or more.

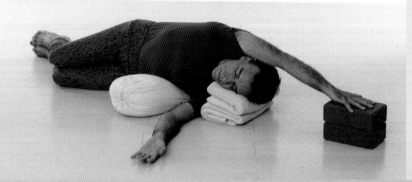

what to do while you're there

As you rest in each position, enjoy the way the inhalation seems to move more into the top lung. If you are lying on your left side, let the right side of the torso swell with each inhalation and visualize the right lung filling with fresh air, bringing good pranic energy into your system. The left side of your torso will press down into the support with each inhalation, so enjoy the

2. Move the brick backward by 12cm (5in) and take your right arm back with it, so that your palm still rests on it. At this stage you are still in a pure side-stretch, so don't change the torso positioning. Stay for two minutes, or more if you are loving it.

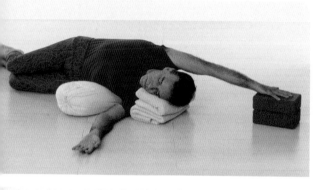

3. Now move the brick backward approximately another 25cm (10in). This time you'll bring your torso into a twist, so that your heart opens more to the sky. Allow your face to turn upward just the right amount, and turn your palm up, too. Adjust for comfort and stay for another two minutes. Then turn around, ready to move through the three stages on your right side.use your hand to help bring one thigh up and slowly roll out to the side.

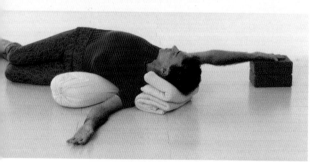

massaging effects this has on the muscles of the left side. Imagine that this slow, rhythmic massage is even soothing your organs, too.

take care

Don't stay in the pose if feels uncomfortable. Activate your stretched muscles before you move to come out of the pose.

☆ child poses

Many people find these postures soothing for the brain as well as the back. Enjoy turning your back on the world as you rest and travel inward during Child Pose.

basic child pose

This version is most commonly used during active Hatha yoga practice to take a rest break, either short or long.

Kneel with your knees together. Sit back on your heels and fold forward to rest your forehead on the floor. Drape your arms beside your legs, palms up. Allow your shoulders to roll in. Adjust as required. Some people prefer their head turned to one side, in which case do alternate between left and right. If your forehead doesn't touch the floor, try bringing your arms forward to make a little shelf for your forehead with one or two stacked fists; again, let the shoulders slouch happily.

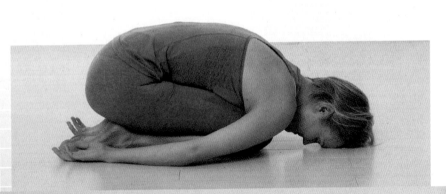

what to do while you're there

Child Pose is a great opportunity to explore breathing into the different parts of the torso. In all three of these Child Poses, movement of the breath into the front of your body is restricted (by either the thighs or the soft support), offering the invitation to breathe into the back of the body. Soften the back of the heart as your back muscles release with each inhalation. Enjoy how the wave of each inhalation subtly increases the pressure

supported child pose

This asymmetrical option helps reset the breathing to a slow and steady rate, even long after your practice.

elevated child pose

Enjoy feeling a lovely length through your front body, as you fill your body with breath and light while relaxing to the max.

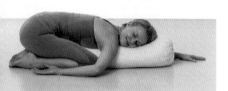

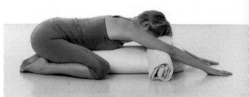

Kneel with your big toes touching and your knees wide apart. Take a bolster or folded-up blankets between your thighs and lay your torso down. Some people need two bolsters to keep the spine in a restful horizontal line. To enjoy a passive release along the side of the torso, reach your left arm forward, resting your forearm to the floor, while your right arm drapes back. Turn your head to figure out which cheek it feels nicest to rest on. Close your eyes and enjoy the sense of your left lung inflating with fresh air, filling your torso with lightness. Stay for one to five minutes, then change to side two.

Fold a blanket to create a firm roll about 10cm (4in) thick. Place it near the top of a bolster to form a T-shape. With feet together, but knees wide, lay your belly and chest down on the bolster. Reach your arms forward, to rest the area around your elbows on top of the roll. Bring your forehead to rest on the edge of the roll. You want to ensure that the height and position are right, so that your nose is clear to breathe easily (with a light tucking in of your chin) and your neck feels comfortable in the slightly flattened position. Placing the forehead on a yoga brick placed in front of the roll works for many. The heightened position of the armpits allows the shoulders to release while your chest sinks deliciously into the bolster. Stay here for a minute or ten!

on the belly and chest, and sense how pleasant the reliable, soothing breath is as the pressure on the abdominal organs gently increases and decreases like a soothing massage.

take care

Don't stay in the pose if feels uncomfortable. Activate your stretched muscles before you move to come out of the pose, and use your arm strength to bring you up.

CHILD POSES

backbend ripple

Doesn't the name of this restorative posture sound like a yummy summer-berry ice cream? And, for your body, it tastes just as good. Only, as it's so good for you, there's no need for any guilt as you linger there a while. Your spine will thank you for tasting this pose – so go on and lap it up.

1. Roll up a blanket to form a roll about 70cm (27in) long x 9cm (3½in) high and place it crossways on the floor. This will go under your back and is the most important element. If you have more props handy, use them to add these next two elements. Take a bolster, or roll up two more blankets to 15cm (6in) high, to place under your knees. Take another blanket or large towel and roll it up to half the height of your knee support, about 7cm (3in). This will go under the Achilles curves, between your calves and heels.

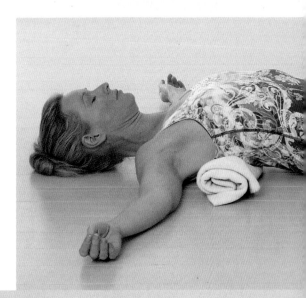

what to do while you're there
Practise the Rectangular Breath (see page 334) or, a little more challenging, Square Breathing: exhale to empty the lungs, then inhale to fill them for a count of four. Hold your breath in for four beats, then exhale to empty for four beats. Hold your breath out for a count of four. Do three rounds in total; they can be consecutive or you can take some recovery breaths in between. Then relax completely.

2. Put your knee and ankle supports in place. Then lie down so that the back roll is positioned at the midpoint of your ribcage, just under the armpits. Take your arms out wide, palms up. If it feels better, release more into the shoulders by taking them closer to the ears to form a Y-shape. Your neck should feel long and graceful. If your chin is in the air and your throat feels open and vulnerable, that's a sign that your neck is too arched. Either reduce the size of the back roll or fold another blanket under the head to elevate it slightly. Hold for two to ten minutes. Then remove the back roll and lie flat. Marvel at how lusciously long and elegantly flat your back feels.

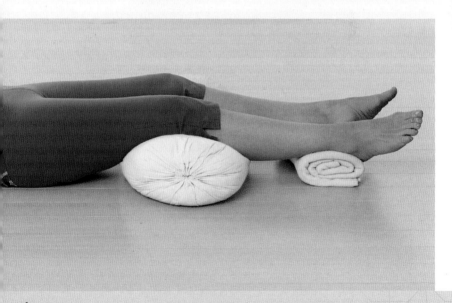

take care
Don't stay in this pose if it feels uncomfortable. Activate your stretched muscles before you move to come out of the pose. Start with a shorter stay and extend it over several practices. Don't lie on your back in pregnancy after 14 weeks.

☆ restorative twists

While restorative yoga postures can feel incredibly gentle, profound changes can occur. Don't underestimate the power of taking some time in these supported shapes.

side-lying *savasana*

As many of the muscles that help you breathe get a stretch, being supremely supported in this pose, it means that your breathing can slow and steady.

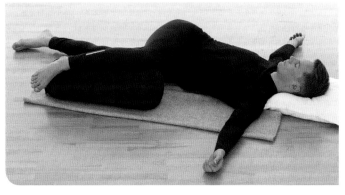

Start by lying on a soft surface on your left side. If you have plenty of props, snuggle a bolster or rolled blankets alongside your spine. Bend your right knee up level with your right hip. Support the leg from the right knee to the foot with a bolster or more blankets, folded as high as your right hip joint. Use a small cushion or folded blanket to lift your head up, so that the neck follows the line and height of the rest of the spine. Extend your right arm away behind you. Once you know how high your right shoulder naturally sits, place blankets folded to shoulder height under the entire length of the arm. Some people won't need any support under the back arm at all. Choose the position for your neck and head that feels best for you. Rest for two to five minutes. Then practise the second side.

what to do while you're there

Most twists, restorative or not, will tend to feel as if they close down the breathing a little on one side. If you twist toward the left, the expansion of the left side of the ribs feels constricted, as if you have to work harder to breathe deeply into that left lung. On the other hand, it's easy and natural to enhance the expansion on the right side. As you rest in your twists, observe this

simple restorative twist

So supportive, so soothing – let your body soak up the benefits of this one.

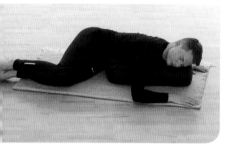

Sit with a bolster (or blankets folded to a bolster shape) placed end on next to your left hip. Bend your knees in, so that both feet are near the right hip. Twist your torso to the left and place one hand on either side of your prop. Push into the floor to increase the twist and better line up your chestbone, which should be centred to the bolster. Then slide the hands forward, to rest your chest and belly down on the support. Check that your elbows are forward of the shoulders, and wide enough to really allow the shoulders to slump in happy relaxation. Try out which direction you prefer to face: forward or back. Stay for up to five minutes. Then repeat on the second side.

restorative eagle twist

Enjoy the lovely outer hip and thigh release this twist offers.

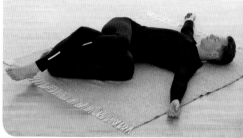

Lie on your back with a bolster to your left, placed from hip to knee. Bend both knees and wrap your right thigh around the left. If you can, entwine the right foot behind the left calf. Place the feet on the floor, lift your hips and move your buttocks 5cm (2in) to the right. Then lift the feet up again. Activate your abdominal muscles and slowly lower your legs to rest on the bolster. If this feels too strong, raise the height of your support. If you have lower-back issues, unravel your legs and rest them on the support, right leg on top of left leg, with knees bent. Close your eyes and breathe here for two to four minutes. Separate the legs before bringing them up one at a time to get ready for side two.

phenomenon, and delight in expanding into the freer side. When you come to the second side, the contracted side will have its turn, too, so it will all even out for you.

take care

Seek further advice before trying these restorative twists if you have any tendency toward sacroiliac dysfunction, a slipped (herniated) disc or lower-back pain.

☆ resting pigeon

Allowing the front leg to drop to a lower plane takes the edge off the classic Pigeon Pose and elevates it into the restorative yoga category that many find it easier to relax into.

1. Position two bolsters so that they initially form one long line. If you don't have yoga bolsters, make two wedges using two to four blankets each. How many you need will depend on their size and thickness, and you may enjoy a higher wedge more if you need to accommodate sore knees, tight hips or a heavier body. Fold up each blanket to form a wedge approximately 80 x 30 x 15cm (30 x 12 x 6in).

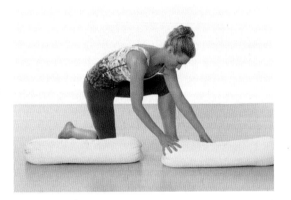

2. Move the top bolster about 10cm (4in) to the left. Then make a space between them of about 30cm (12in). Bring your right knee into the space in between, and just out to the right side of the front bolster. Take your right ankle close to the left side of the bottom bolster.

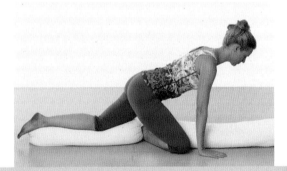

what to do while you're there

Practice *bhramari* (buzzing bee) breathing, to calm the nervous system: breathe in and out through the nose and, each time you exhale, make a buzzing sound like a bee. This will encourage your exhalations to lengthen out, in an incredibly restful way. Be sure to relax during each inhalation as well, to counterbalance each long, slow exhalation. Practise this breathing

3. Rest your left thigh, knee and shin on the bottom bolster. Slide your left leg back and away, to lower your hips and find a gentle stretch in your right buttock. Lay your torso down on the front bolster, ensuring that it's easy to relax your belly and chest into the softness of the support. Take your elbows out wide, so that you can fully give the weight of your forearms to the floor. Slide them slightly forward of the shoulder line, to find the best shoulder release, and take them wide. Turn your head in both directions to test which cheek you prefer to rest on, or stay for half your allotted time on each. Close your eyes and rest for five minutes before changing to the second side. Keep warm with a soft cover, if required.

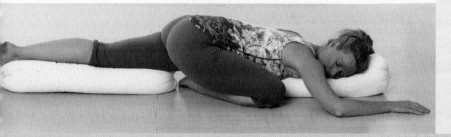

for the first half of the time you spend in Resting Pigeon, then fall into silence for the remainder, enjoying the soothing vibration that is moving through your body.

take care
This option suits many who can't manage other Pigeon variations due to knee issues. Even so, ensure your bent knee feels supremely comfortable and pain-free during your practice, and seek advice where necessary.

restorative forward bends

Use any combination of props to create the most comfortable support for you. Various bolster, blanket and chair combinations are shown below, so experiment to find your favourite. As the body releases while you hold the posture, push the props away a little, to deepen the pose. Keep the intensity level low. Remember: with restorative postures, allow time – rather than intensity – to do the work for you.

resting head-beyond-the-knee pose

Sit on the front edge of a folded blanket about 5cm (2in) high to assist the anterior tilt at the pelvis. Bend your right knee out to the right and snuggle the sole of the foot to the left inner thigh. Place one or more bolsters crossways over your left leg. Fold forward to rest your arms and forehead on your bolster (or use a chair, as shown in the Resting Wide-Leg Releases, opposite). Be sure your nose is clear, so that you can breathe easily. Use an extra-soft block or blanket to lift the forehead if you feel the head drops too low. Hold for two minutes on each side. Stay present, and nudge the props away once you feel that the body can accept more stretch.

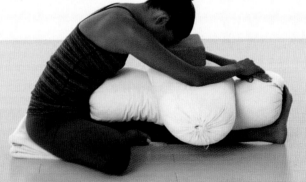

what to do while you're there

Enjoy soft belly-breathing. So often we hold tightness where we just don't need to. Scan over your body and allow all your muscles to deactivate, so that any unnecessary holding can release. Imagine that by resting the forehead you are giving the whole frontal lobe of your brain a rest, too.

RESTORATIVE YOGA

restorative double-leg stretch

Sit on the edge of a folded blanket, with both legs stretched out in front. Lay a bolster lengthways along your legs, and fold forward to rest your belly and chest on it. If your torso doesn't touch the prop, stack a long folded blanket on top, to a height where you are supported. You might prefer to use a chair, as shown in the Resting Wide-Leg Releases. Fold another blanket across your supports, so that you can rest your forehead at a height where the neck follows the natural line of the spine. The light pressure of the forehead against the support becomes an important part of the restfulness of these forward bends. Keeping the arms up higher than floor level helps to open the front of the body, which aids effective breathing. Stay for two to four minutes.

resting wide-leg releases

Sit on the front edge of a folded blanket 5cm (2in) high. Bring the soles of the feet together, so that the knees bend out wide. Bring your heels toward your hips. Tilting forward from the pelvis, reach your arms forward and bring them over the seat of a chair. Have the chair far enough away that you feel a gentle stretch in the inner thighs, back or buttocks – or all of these points. Rest your head on the padded front edge of the chair seat. Using a yoga block can help if you are dropping the head too far for comfort. If you don't feel any stretch at all, try taking the pose lower, by using bolsters and folded blankets, as shown in the other two photos. Stay for two to four minutes. Next, try a supported wide-legged pose, with both legs extended out wide in a V-shape.

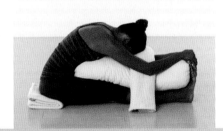 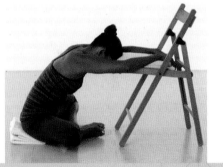

RESTORATIVE FORWARD BENDS

take care
Avoid these forward bends in cases of a slipped (herniated) disc or sacroiliac dysfunction.

restorative inversion – legs up the wall

More than a yoga pose, this inversion is known as a *mudra*, a mood-altering pose that is believed to benefit the flow of *prana*, or life energy, through the whole body. So simple, so delicious. Ten or so minutes in this resting version of Shoulder-Stand will change the tone of your whole day.

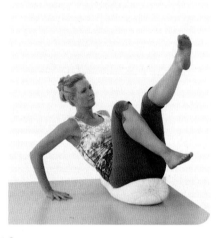

1. Take a yoga bolster, or fold a blanket to about 80 x 30 x 15cm (30 x 12 x 6in), and place it around 15cm (6in) from a wall. Sit on the bolster, sideways to the wall, so that one hip and shoulder tip touch the wall. Take your arms to the floor behind you and lean back. Swivel on your buttocks as you bring your legs up the wall – if it feels too awkward, try moving the bolster a little further away on the floor.

2. As your legs come up, you can rest your shoulders and head down on the floor. Check your alignment: your sacrum should be on the support; your lower back should drape over the bolster edge; your tailbone (which may be close to the wall or further away if you are less flexible) should be on the wall side of the bolster. Your chin, chestbone, pubic bone and big toes should be in a line. Most importantly, you should feel supremely

what to do while you're there

Count yourself deeper into stillness. Start at 27 and track your breath, by mentally repeating: "I am breathing in 27. I am breathing out 27. I am breathing in 26. I am breathing out 26." And so on, down to one. If you lose count, return to 27 and start again. Don't get tense about this – the aim is not necessarily to reach one. The aim is simply to focus, slow your mind and stay present. If you

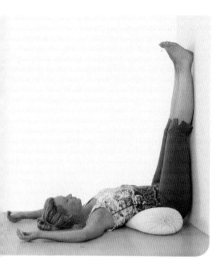
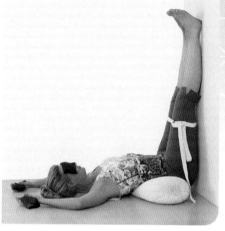

comfortable. Stay for at least five minutes and up to 15. To come out, bend your knees and press your feet into the wall. Slide your bolster to the side, then lower your hips back down and roll out to the side. After several breaths, use your arms to push yourself up to sitting.

3. Consider the following options to help you relax in this pose. Take a soft belt and tie it around your mid-thighs; this will enable your leg muscles to fully release from the effort of subtly keeping the legs together. Place a light covering on your eyes. To help those ever-busy hands surrender to stillness, place a light weight like an eye-pillow in each palm. You will continue to cool down as you rest, particularly with your feet up high, so be sure to stay warm: cover yourself from the feet down with a soft blanket.

reach one, then your mind will be trained on your breath. You will be in meditation and can continue to follow the breaths with no further need to count.

take care

If you are menstruating, practise this pose without the bolster so that your upper body rests entirely on the floor. In pregnancy, don't practise it after 35 weeks.

ancient wisdom for modern life: your true nature

PARUŚA पुरुष

Yoga philosophy encompasses other Vedantic philosophies, one of the primary ones being *Samkhya*. According to *Samkhya*, there are two primary life forces: matter and that which animates it. *Puruśa* is the aspect of our being that has a higher unchanging consciousness. As it is pure consciousness, *puruśa* is the higher Self. It is completely free of ego. It is constant and unchanging in humans and in the universe. Being beyond subject or object, the concept of *puruśa* can be tricky to grasp, because it's beyond the mind and it cannot be made to be an object, as it is the very source of perception. *Puruśa* is pure consciousness. It is eternal, indestructible, without form and all-pervasive.

The partner of *puruśa*, which impacts on everything we do, is *prakriti*. *Prakriti*

PRAKRITI प्रकृति

प्रकृति

is the tangible, perceivable, material reality. This includes things we may not be able to see, such as infrared light or the sound waves responsible for mobile technology. It is the aspect of everything that is subject to cause and effect. Unlike *puruśa*, which is unchanging in humans and the universe, *prakriti* is subject to change. You can think of *prakriti* as matter and of *puruśa* as spirit. *Pakriti* relates to

your (small "s") self-identity and is very tied up in ego. Without the constant existence of *puruśa* in the background, *prakriti* could not exist. Unlike *puruśa*, which has an eternal quality, the defining quality of *prakriti* is that it is subject to change. The consciousness of *puruśa* animates *prakriti*, giving life to all forms of matter, such as nature, animals and human beings.

ARE WE SEPARATE OR ONE?

A fundamental cause of our suffering is that we confuse *puruśa* and *prakriti*. On a practical basis, we assume an identity to navigate life experience, and in the process this causes us to forget who we truly are. This creates a feeling of being separate from our innate interconnection with the entire universe.

Separateness is our experience. It is valid; it is real to us and cannot be denied. But it's a relative separateness, because our other reality is oneness. As we exist with two concurrent realities, we tend to suffer as we mistake our (small "s") self-identity, *prakriti*, with our true and pure (capital "S") Self, *puruśa*. We need somehow to accept that we are both separate and one.

When the mind is clear, we come to know our true Self. With a highly refined mind, we experience the nature of *puruśa*. The path to one leads to an understanding of the other. When we come to know *puruśa*, we come to know ourselves. Likewise, when we come to know ourselves, we come to know *puruśa*.

SO EXACTLY WHO ARE YOU?

The teachings of yoga remind us that we are not our role, job title, what we do, what we do well, our spreadsheet, our mission statement or our values list. We are also more than man/woman, son/daughter, worker/colleague, mother/father, sister/brother or lover/fighter. We are pure and beyond all these categories. We just are.

To focus on this idea and help you identify with the ultimate reality, try repeating "*So Ham*" as you sit in meditation. *So Ham* means "I am that". On each inhalation, mentally repeat, "*So*"; on each exhalation, repeat, "*Ham*".

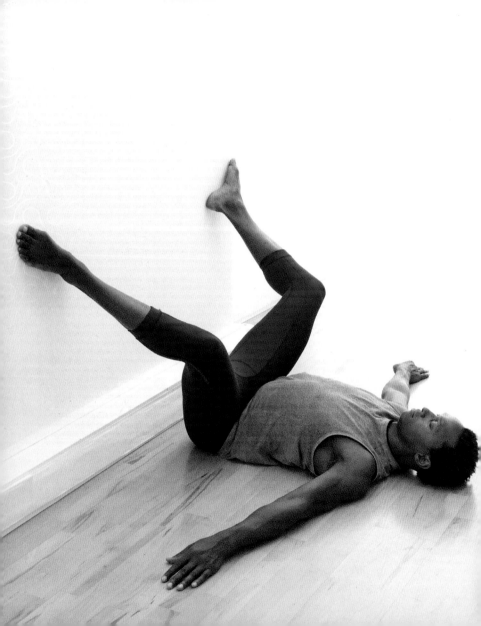

15

YIN YOGA

At its heart, yin yoga is a meditative practice. It's a time when you allow yourself to open. With plenty of time to contemplate, you'll cultivate mindfulness, bringing your attention to the present experience. This witnessing of the stream of consciousness will actively dissipate any build-up of stress. It will allow you to feel lighter and more joyful.

The slow yin poses in this section are the perfect antidote to the general fast pace at which we conduct our modern lives. They are a great counterbalance to the active yang-yoga practices, and to any other fast-moving exercise you may enjoy, and this is why yin yoga has grown in popularity around the world over the past few years.

While an energy-raising (active Hatha) yoga practice is useful to help us complete our daily tasks, we do need an aspect where we can simply let ourselves open. Transformation occurs when you become still, quiet and open to listening. Yin uses your body as an instrument, and the postures as your tools to transformation and transcendence. Each yin posture comes with a precious gift for you – the opportunity for exploration of the Self. With regular yin practice, you are guaranteed a better understanding of the mind–body connection, as this introspective practice links and harmonizes your body, mind, heart and soul. Over time you will see yourself more clearly, become familiar with any habitual patterning of the mind and, in doing so, create some space for simply being. (Remember: first you are a human *being*, before you are a human *doing*.) Then you can become open and free. Try it out – what have you got to lose?

How does yin yoga work?

Yin yoga poses apply moderate and appropriate stress to the bones, synovial capsules and other connective tissues of the body: the tendons, ligaments and fascia. These tissues are considered to have yin qualities – being cool, binding, slow-changing, passive and immobile – when compared to the muscles that are considered yang. The yang nature is warm, elastic, faster-changing, active and mobile.

The goal of yin yoga is to nourish the connective tissue, improve circulation and flexibility in the joints, and ensure them a good supply of synovial fluid. Each of the yin yoga postures works with one or more of the Chinese energy meridians, or channels, and the aim of yin yoga is to improve the flow of *chi* (energy), not only in the joints, but also through these energy channels.

During yin yoga, static postures are held for around two to five minutes each, or sometimes longer. This is distinct from the "yang", or active, yoga styles, which have comparatively shorter holds and feature movement and repetition.

When we exercise muscles, they weaken, then repair and rebuild themselves, becoming stronger. So we know that some physical stress is actually a good thing, and that the human body can masterfully adapt to it. Similarly, it's not good news when a joint is not placed under physical stress. If a joint is immobilized long term (such as in a plaster cast), it will "freeze" and degenerate. The body welcomes and needs a certain amount of physical stress to remain strong and flexible.

Yin tissues are best exercised in a yin way, and yang tissues in a yang way. The mobile and elastic yang tissues, such as your muscles, love movement and muscular engagement. However, if you were to work your muscles in the slow yin way – say, by tensing a muscle group for five minutes – uncomfortable contraction, cramping and soreness would result. Nor does it always work well to exercise your yin tissues in an overly yang way. For example, fast, strong, repetitive weightlifting can be too aggressive for the joints and can cause injury. Think of the teeth, which, being fairly immobile, are considered to be yin tissues. You wouldn't attempt to change a child's bite with a sudden, dramatic wrench on their teeth. Instead, orthodontists use braces to apply a constant pressure, sustained over a long time, to realign children's teeth. Yin yoga operates in a similar way, using a constant pressure and the longer holds of several minutes each. Therefore the magic of yin lies in consistent, appropriate physical stress (not stretch), combined with time.

YIN YOGA

306

When can I practise yin yoga?

You can practise daily, if you balance yin yoga with other active and strengthening exercise. Keep in mind than yin yoga is not a complete practice by itself. It targets the lower body a little more than the upper, and it won't make your muscles strong or your heart beat faster. Yin is a perfect complement to active (yang) yoga practices, and to any other active exercise you enjoy. A once-a-week complete yin practice will nicely counterbalance a regular active yoga practice or other sporting pursuits.

If you'd like to do a full yin practice, follow the poses in this section in the order they are given, and finish with a Simple Restorative Twist (see page 292), followed by any of the practices from the "Relaxations to Revel In" section (see pages 346–59) and some time in seated Mindfulness Meditation (see page 366). You might book-end your regular yoga practice with a yin pose or two, rotating them over time, to cycle through a selection. Yin yoga is a great evening practice for insomniacs and a helpful lead-in to relaxation and meditation. Of course, if you are injured, do seek advice from an expert before you practice. While props are less often used in yin yoga than in restorative yoga, do use padding to add softness as required.

What should I be feeling?

The yin way of exercise is to use a slow, sustained pressure. The aim is to protect the joints, nourish them and build mobility, while keeping them safe as you apply a therapeutic stress though them. So while yin postures place stress through the yin tissues of the body, it should be a *healthy* and *appropriate* stress, within your natural range of motion for that joint. Intuitively things should feel okay; you need to have an emotional willingness to stay in the posture. The physical focus shifts to the connective tissue, rather than feeling it in the muscles or tendons. While you expect to feel a certain slow tensioning, you definitely want to avoid uncomfortable compression. There will be no brief, jerky, bouncy or explosive stretch.

You might choose to practise your yin postures with an intensity of anywhere from three to eight, on a scale of ten. Most likely there will be slowly undulating waves of intensity, with a sense of build-ups and releases. Thoughts and impressions will come to you, so use them as a reminder to practise mindfulness. As you stay in the postures, you will have time for introspection and release, and can develop your awareness of the inner silence.

try this out

Engage your finger and palm muscles to actively stretch out the fingers of one hand. Take one fingertip between two fingers of the other hand and pull on it. Most likely you won't feel any difference in the reach or lengthening in that finger. Now soften the muscles of the hand, and again, pull on that fingertip. When the muscles are disengaged, you will feel a sense of "give" in the joints. There is some lengthening, and space is being created. This is the feeling you are aiming for in your yin poses. With your muscles deactivated, the work can begin on the joints.

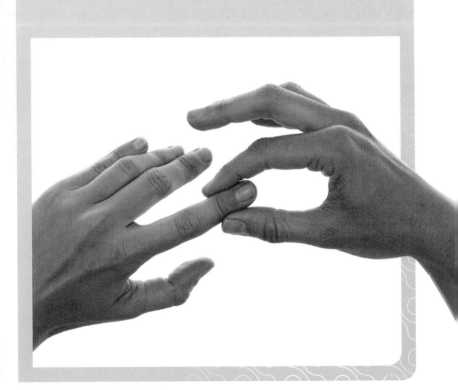

Guidelines to your yin practice

- **You need to enter the postures slowly**, so that the body feels safe to release and won't tighten up in resistance. You might need to move a little at first, in order to settle into stillness. Then be still.

- **Work with soft muscles** to shift the focus to working with the joints. When the muscles are tight around a joint, the joint capsule won't take on the load (healthy stress), which is the aim of yin yoga. If you have hyper-mobile joints, avoid pushing into them and learn to develop more sensitivity at their edge.

- **Yin yoga should not be painful**, although it is character-building and you can expect to feel waves of intensity. If you are feeling pain, don't work so deeply into the posture and find ways to increase the support, such as padding under the body. Speak with a yin-yoga teacher to ensure you are on the right track. Take it easy if you have injuries, and use props where necessary.

- **Tiptoe toward your "edge"**, so that you come to an appropriate edge within any natural range of motion. There is no aesthetic ideal in yin yoga. It needs to feel safe to you. Only *you* are on the inside of your experience, so only you can know that for yourself. As with active yoga, from moment to

moment, day to day and practice to practice, your edges will be different. Be sensible and sensitive.

- **Stay a while.** Be still at that edge, with an attitude of surrendering into the shape and sensations. Cultivate awareness and curiosity. Dissolve any of your preferences. Let your awareness shine a light for you. You might hold some poses for just one minute, so be content with that.

- **Assume a neutral position** after each pose. Lie on your back in between yin postures, to allow the *chi* energy to circulate.

- **A little bit of courage is needed** to effect change. You need to sit at your edge in order for the shifts to happen. If you don't push those boundaries, things will tend to stay the same.

- **Open to calm abiding.** Long holds in the short term create discomfort, resentment and resistance. There may be uncomfortable feelings of being stuck – anything but being open and free. Remember that these states of mind and body aren't permanent. However, we tend to perceive them as permanent, and that's where we fall into struggle. Remind yourself that it's not about finding a mood, but rather about existing in a quality of the mind that incorporates all moods.

butterfly

This posture stretches the lines of energy along the inner and outer legs. It works along the liver and kidney meridians at the inner thighs, on the gall-bladder at the outer thighs, and on the urinary-bladder meridian at the back. This pose supports the healthy functioning of the reproductive system, the prostate for men, and is useful for women during pregnancy.

1. Take a blanket and fold it up several layers thick. Sitting on the edge of your blanket, bring the soles of the feet together in front of you and take your knees out wide. Place your feet further away than your knees to create a diamond shape with your legs.

what to do while you're there

The intensity will wax and wane as you hold each pose. While it's your responsibility to yourself to ensure you are not hurting your bones, joints or muscles in yoga, it is normal for the intensity to shift, even as you hold the same pose. Observe how you respond to these intensities, and develop a sense of detachment. Practise being the silent witness to your experience, to neutralize reactions that make your thoughts jump around.

how to come out

Press yourself upright. Use your hands to help bring your knees up, and place your feet flat on the floor in front of you. Lean back on your hands and lift your hips in the air. Then lower down. Repeat several times. With feet and buttocks on the floor, take both knees to one side, then the other side, in a style similar to Reclining Eagle Twist (see page 226).

2. Take your fingertips to the floor in front of you. Tilting from the hips, tip forward until you feel the beginnings of a pull on your muscles. Allow the head to hang down. Then move one more notch forward, until your spine moves from a flat to a rounded shape and you find your first "edge" – a holding point that is no more than six out of ten on the scale of intensity. Three minutes is a a good length of time to for at the start, and you can build this up to eight over repeated practices. (Setting an alarm is helpful during yin postures.) Maintain a light supportive pressure through the arms. Over time, you might walk your hands forward, or even bring your elbows to the floor. If your head comes all the way to the floor, take it inside your heels rather than beyond your toes. Take the intensity up to seven out of ten for the last minute, or eight for a few breaths just before your time is up.

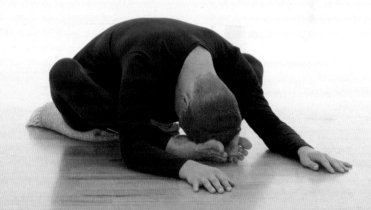

modifications and cautions

Take care if you have sciatica. Try raising the hips on a much higher prop, such as a firm cushion or bolster, or avoid this pose altogether. Avoid dropping the head down if you have had neck issues. You could try supporting the forehead on a long, high bolster to keep the neck in its natural neutral curve. If you have any slipped (herniated) disc issues, you need to avoid rounding the back at all. Instead, practise this pose lying down – try out the Yin Happy Baby on page 318 or Resting Cobbler's Poses on page 284. As with all yin postures, if you experience any harmful sensations, such as sharp, hot or stabbing pains, come out of the pose. Before practising this pose, read the "Guidelines to your yin practice" on page 309.

sphinx and seal

These two backbends can be a real gift to your lower back. Start off with a shorter hold and build up once you know how your body responds.

sphinx

The Sphinx is your starter option, before moving on to the Seal. The backbend shape works into the urinary-bladder and kidney meridians.

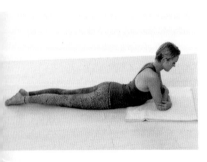

1. Place a folded blanket where your forearms will be. Lie on the floor and, with your arms out in front, bend each elbow to cup it in the opposite hand. Curve your back into a backbend, starting with your elbows a little forward of the shoulder line. If that feels too strong for your back, move them forward a notch or two. In yin, your holding point is where the muscles are not switched on, so enjoy getting slouchy through your shoulders. Remember: you want to deactivate the muscles to take the work to the joints.

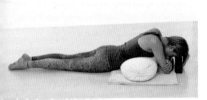

2. Choose whether you would like to keep the neck in a neutral forward position, allow the head to hang down or rest your forehead on a yoga brick. Let your legs find their natural width apart. If it feels too strong, put a yoga bolster under the belly to support the abdomen. Stay for up to three to five minutes.

what to do while you're there

If the intensity is too strong for you in either pose, try activating the back muscles to do an engaged version of the pose for short pockets of time. Then soften into the yin pose for a bit. This way, you can move in and out of softness.

how to come out

Lie flat. When you are ready, lift yourself to kneel on all fours. Exhale and take the hips back toward the heels in Basic Child Pose (see page 288). Then inhale to return to all fours. Continue moving between these two positions for several rounds. In Child Pose again, move the hips from side to side. Reclining Twist Flow (see page 40) is lovely after these backbends.

seal

This stronger posture has the same benefits as the Sphinx. It gives an additional stomach stretch, plus deeper actions on the stomach and spleen meridians.

From Sphinx, walk your hands forward and take them wider apart. Lift your elbows to straighten your arms, which will prop you up, stilt-like. With your elbows locked, choose your level of intensity – whether you want to walk your hands closer to the body or further away. Disengage your back and buttock muscles. While a small amount of compression may stimulate energy stagnation in the lower back, ensure you don't overdo it: check that you are feeling tension, more than a compression, through the spine. Allow the shoulders to sag. Stay for up to one to five minutes. Initially you can build up to this by holding for periods of 30 seconds with short rests in between.

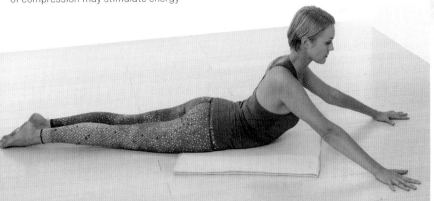

modifications and cautions

Avoid during pregnancy, if you have lower-back compression, sacral discomfort or conditions where you shouldn't perform spinal extension. Come out, if you experience back pain or headache. Before practising this pose, read the "Guidelines to your yin practice" on page 309.

yin child and child with a twist

These two restful postures can feel deeply healing. They also feel great after a backbend.

yin child

This pose works into the joints of the spine and the hips, while the kidney and urinary-bladder meridians get a rebalance.

Kneel on a padded surface. Bring your big toes together and widen your knees apart. Sit your hips back as close as possible toward your heels. Walk both hands as far forward as possible, allowing your chest to drop toward the floor. Rest your forehead on the floor. Let go of any muscle working in this pose. As the back muscles deactivate, the work in the joints can begin. Allow a sense of melting to come. Stay for three to five minutes. Come out, or move on to Yin Child with a Twist.

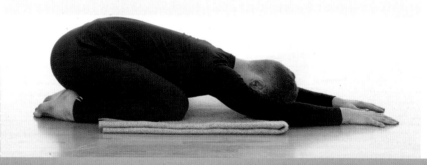

what to do while you're there

Imagine that any pockets of discomfort are as large as the entire space you are practising in, so that they dilute. As they diffuse and diminish, open to the experience of ease. You can also use conscious breathing to dissolve the intensity. Breathe into where you feel it most, then allow each exhalation to scoop it out your body so that you become hollow. Each exhalation can empty out those strong sensations.

how to come out

Walk your hands in and push yourself up to kneeling. Take a Starter Headstand (see page 264) for five or ten breaths. Then lie on your back in Corpse Pose (see pages 348–52), with your limbs stretched out wide, and absorb the shifts in your energies as a result of this posture.

yin child with a twist

This version has all the benefits of the Yin Child, while the shoulder-release allows the stretch to work into the heart and lung meridians.

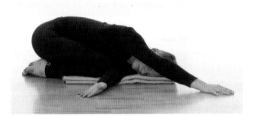

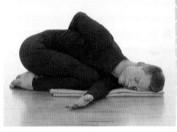

1. From your starter Yin Child pose, walk your hands in to come up a little. Walk both hands toward the right and position one hand on either side of your right knee. With your hips still back and down, and both arms outreached, thread your left arm through the window of the right arm, ensuring it clears your right knee. Settle your left shoulder on the floor near your right knee. Turn your head to the right and lay it to rest on the floor. Progress on to step 2, or hold here for two to three minutes before working into the second side.

2. Wrap your right arm around your lower back to hook your hand onto the front of the left hip. If you can't reach, hold onto your waistband. Let your right arm and shoulder go heavy as the muscles release. Stay here for two or three minutes. Then practise side two.

modifications and cautions

Take care if you have any groin, hip or back problems, as this pose may not be for you. Place padding under the knees or ankles, if required. If your knees don't like this pose, try placing a folded blanket between your seat and ankles, so that they don't need to bend as much. Placing a bolster under the chest makes this pose feel easier. If your hips don't come close to your heels, take some support – such as a yoga brick – under the forehead. All yoga poses need to feel safe while you are in them, so come up without delay if you feel unsafe. Before practising this pose, read over the "Guidelines to your yin practice" on page 309.

shoelace

This deep hip release lengthens the lower back to relieve tension there. It works along the liver meridian at the inner thigh, and along the gall-bladder meridian of the outer thigh and hip.

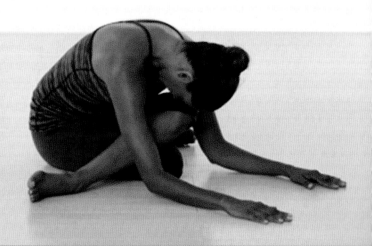

what to do while you're there

Check that you are not striving, forcing or pushing. As you hold the poses with your muscles deactivated as much as possible, you will experience phases of release. Your hip joints and vertebral joints will respond to these long holds over time. Practise mindfulness – be present to just where you are in the moment.

how to come out

Come out of all yin postures slowly. Use your arms to push yourself upright. Unravel your legs and bend them in front of you. With feet flat on the floor, lift your hips in the air a few times to form a table-like shape. Then lie on your back, with your feet on the floor and your knees bent, and move both legs to one side and then the other, like windscreen wipers.

1. If you are new to this practice, sit your hips up on a cushion or folded blanket. From a cross-legged position, move your knees toward each other, until one stacks on top of the other. Usually each foot will snuggle near an outer hip at the beginning stages. However, if your hips are naturally more flexible, you might move each foot a little wider out and a bit further forward. If your hips are tighter, then try the Half Shoelace: straighten the bottom leg all the way out in front. This is also useful if you experience pain in the bottom knee.

2. Whether you are in Half or Full Shoelace, tilt forward from the hips and take your hands to the floor in front, placing them on either side of your knees. If your spine is still straight, walk your hands forward until it starts to round and you feel a slight pull by the outer hips or in the back. At this starting point, allow the head to hang forward and rest. Check that the intensity level is around six out of ten, or less if necessary.

3. Set your arms up for the long hold of this yin pose. You can rest your elbows on your top leg, or it can feel nice to bend your elbows to rest your forehead on your palms. Some people enjoy leaning in and resting the forehead on a prop, such as a bolster standing on its end, or foam yoga blocks. Others are able to take their elbows all the way to the floor. If you try this, keep in mind that the aim of this yin pose is not to feel a strong stretch in the muscles, but rather to place a controlled and appropriate stress through the connective tissues of the body.

4. Start with a three-minute hold and build up to five minutes. In the last minute you may increase the intensity to seven out of ten, then eight for the final breaths. Follow the "how to come out" guidelines before practising the second side.

modifications and cautions

Avoid the Shoelace pose if you suffer from sciatica. Avoid hanging your head down if you have had neck issues. You could try supporting the forehead on a long, high bolster to keep the neck in its natural neutral curve. If you have any slipped (herniated) disc issues, you need to avoid rounding the back at all – you could lie on your back, cross your bent legs at your thighs and hug both legs in. If you have knee pain in Shoelace, you could put padding under the top knee to lift it. As with all yin postures, if you experience pain, come out of the pose or back off until it dissipates. Before practising this pose, read over the "Guidelines to your yin practice" on page 309.

happy baby yin-style

These two postures offer a great
opportunity to work with the pillars
of yin yoga. As you surrender to your
edge, be patient by giving each posture
time, and resolve to practice stillness.

yin happy baby

This strong hip-opener also decompresses
the sacrum. It works on the kidney, urinary-
bladder and liver meridians.

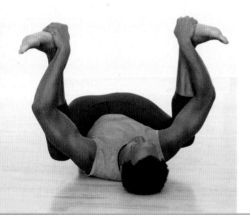

1. Lie on your back. Lift your feet and bend
your knees in toward your armpits. Lift your
head momentarily, as you reach your hands
to the highest point you can grasp. Hold
wherever you can reach: shins, ankles or, if
possible, the insteps of the feet. If that's not
manageable, wrap your palms or forearms
around the backs of your thighs to rest them
there. Let your arms be heavy, which will
help the knees drawing down. Your lower
back will round up, away from the floor.
Rest your head on the floor. Check your
neck alignment. If your chin is lifted and
your throat feels like it's gaping, try to press
the chin toward the throat and lengthen the
neck. If your throat still feels very open, then
place a cushion under the head to better
support the natural curve of the neck. Stay
and breathe for up to three to five minutes.
Observe your breath. Just before coming
out, pull on the legs and widen the feet
apart, to increase the intensity at the hips
for a few breaths.

what to do while you're there

Welcome the sensations of unfolding. Soften your
inner dialogue. There's no rush. Play and surf your
edges. Remember: time is the magic ingredient in
yin practice. Once you reach a more intense state,
stay for one more minute – not with an attitude of
enduring, but instead with an attitude of opening.

how to come out

Cuddle your knees into your chest. Rock
from side to side. If using the wall, slide
away from it, to place both feet on the floor,
with your knees bent. Lift your hips up and
down several times. Then lie flat on your
back, with your limbs stretched out like a
snow angel, and absorb the physical and
energetic shifts in your body.

happy baby using the wall

Many people find this to be a more manageable start to Yin Happy Baby, though when you hold it for long enough, it will still give you those yin-yoga waves of build-up and release.

1. Find a friendly piece of wall and take your legs up it (see page 298 for instructions on getting into position). Bend your knees, to flatten your feet on the wall. Walk your feet apart so that they are a little wider than hip width. Turn your toes out to about 45 degrees, so that the knees also fall away from each other a little. Depending on your flexibility, your sacrum may be lifted off the floor or flat to the floor. To get it down to the floor, ease yourself away from the wall until it touches down. Take your arms wide and a little way up toward the ears to access the upper-body energy meridians. Close your eyes. Once you find an acceptable position, resist the urge to shuffle or move. Rest here for five minutes. Before you come out, grasp the legs or thighs and pull them in, taking a few breaths in Yin Happy Baby.

modifications and cautions

If you are menstruating, keep your sacrum on the floor. Avoid these poses if you have high blood pressure. Before practising these poses, read the "Guidelines to your yin practice" on page 309.

yin dragon lunge

This Dragon Pose works strongly into the hip joint and releases the hip-flexor and quadriceps muscles. It builds mental resilience, as it works all six meridians in the lower half of the body.

1. From an all-fours position, step your right foot between your hands. Take the foot further forward, so that the ankle joint is in front of the knee joint. Still with your hands on the floor, inch your left knee backward as far as possible. With your hands on either side of your front foot, this is your starting Dragon Pose. Lift up to position your hands on your front knee and come into a Flying High Dragon. Check that your lower back feels good here. Remember: with all yin postures, the idea is to strengthen the body by creating an *appropriate* stress in the joints, but not to go into such intensity that there is a feeling of pain.

what to do while you're there

Experienced Hatha yogis who love the movement and flow of active (yang-style) yoga might find that their edge is actually stillness. Our super-busy, high-achieving world doesn't always understand or encourage stillness. A posture where it appears that nothing is happening might present a bit of a challenge to a yogi who is used to the immediate satisfaction of squeezing on strong muscles. If you notice yourself wanting to fidget, or find yourself mentally squirming, what can I say? Be still, rest and trust. Understand that your edge may be stillness and let the pose work its magic.

2. Try out a Flying Low Dragon and see if that's manageable for you. Take your hands to the floor on the left side of your right foot. Walk them forward to lower your elbows to the floor or, if you need a little more height, to a prop such as a folded blanket. Stay in your chosen pose to let everything marinate. Build up to holding your chosen pose for three to five minutes – set a timer, if you like. If you feel it predominantly in the groin, that's the liver and kidney meridians. If the work is more at the front of the thigh of your back leg, the stomach and spleen meridians are being activated. If you feel it more at the outer right thigh, that's the gall-bladder meridian. When your torso is lifted in the Flying High Dragon you may feel it in the lower back, working the urinary, bladder and, again, the kidney meridians.

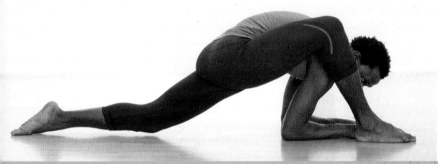

how to come out

Step back to Classic Downward-Facing Dog Pose (see page 58) or Basic Child Pose (see page 288) for several breaths, before coming onto your hands and knees to work into the second side. Reclining Eagle Twist (see page 226) will soften and relax the hips after the intensity of the Dragon.

modifications and cautions

Make it more manageable by placing a support such as a bolster under the back thigh. If your back knee or ankle is uncomfortable, place some soft padding underneath. You could even allow the back knee to float, by placing a folded blanket under the shin. Before practising this pose, read the "Guidelines to your yin practice" on page 309.

yin shoulder stretches

If, as a modern yogi, you feel yourself carrying the weight of the world on your shoulders, these two poses are for you. These deep shoulder releases work into the upper-body meridians to give a good balance to your practice.

criss-cross stretch

I love to breathe into the back of my heart in this pose, feeling it open and blossom. It's nice to shine a light on any tightness there, and allow all those tensions to melt away.

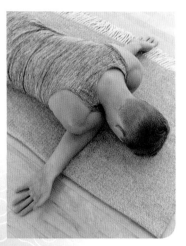

Lie on your front and prop yourself up on your crossed forearms, with the right arm against your chest. Slide your right forearm crossways, thumb up. Reach it to the left, straightening the elbow as much as you can. Then slide your left forearm away to the right. Once it's as straight as it will go, you will find that you can squeeze the right arm straighter, too. Shuffle a little to get your hands one more notch away from each other. Now "walk" your hips forward, to allow your forehead to rest on the floor. Ensure you have come forward enough that your neck is clear, but not so far that your nose compresses to the floor. If you can't reach the floor with ease, rest your forehead on a foam yoga block. Stay for two to three minutes. Then change to the other side.

what to do while you're there

Move your awareness from the external to the internal. Go into the sensations. Experience them as buzzing or vibrations, or as feelings of heat or cold. Sensations tend to break up under scrutiny. Form is not permanent or solid. Don't jump away from seemingly intractable bands of intensity, but instead allow yourself to fall into the subtler sensations, just as you would fall gratefully into a long-awaited and very welcome new season.

yin arm pigeon

This shoulder-opener works into the lung and large-intestine meridians.

Lie on your front, with your left arm stretched straight out to the left side, and the palm level with your shoulder. Turn your head to the right, and place your right palm on the floor close to the right shoulder. Push into your right palm to roll over the left shoulder. Stack your hips. Rest your ear on the floor. Leave your left leg stretched out long, but make it easy to balance by taking your right foot to the floor behind you, knee bent. If you like, wrap your right forearm around your back, tucking it in under your torso. Hold for up to three minutes. Then change to side two.

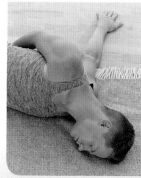

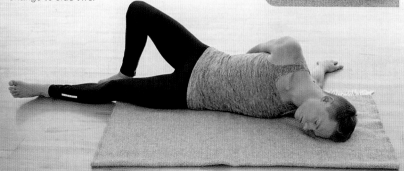

how to come out

Undo the steps to slowly come out. Roll over to lie on your back, with your arms and legs out comfortably wide. Rest a while, enjoying the sensations of release. If you want more for the shoulders, try out Yin Child with a Twist on page 315.

modifications and cautions

Seek advice before practising if you have shoulder troubles. Criss-Cross Stretch is not suitable if you have any conditions where you shouldn't place pressure on the abdomen. Don't practise these poses after ten weeks of pregnancy. Before practising, read the "Guidelines to your yin practice" on page 309.

yin frog

This pose works deeply into the groins and the joints of the hips, lower back and shoulders. It also works on the spleen, liver and kidney meridians. The forward-arm reach involves the heart, lung, and small- and large-intestine meridians.

1. Fold a blanket in half and place it widthways to pad under your knees; or use a cushion under each knee. Start on all fours. Widen out your knees and come down onto your forearms in front of you. Spread your knees apart, keeping them along the same line as your hips, though at the beginning you may find it easier to have your hips slightly forward of the knees. Take your feet away from each other, so that each ankle sits behind the line of its knee. Flex your ankle joints, too, so that your toes point outward. Ultimately this posture is a series of right-angles: at the hips, knees and ankles. For extra comfort, rest your chest on a bolster or folded blanket. Plan to stay for three to five minutes, and read on for a further challenge or a more manageable option.

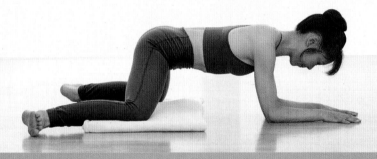

what to do while you're there

When the intensity ramps up, inhale through the nose and sigh out loudly though your mouth. Take three breaths like this, using the exhale to clear out the build-up from your system. Don't let your practice become stressful. Yin yoga aims to mobilize the flow of *chi*, yet stress will inhibit the flow of *chi*. Stay attuned to your emotional willingness to remain in the holds.

how to come out

Depending on how low you are to the ground, you will either slide forward to lie flat on the floor or, with elbows bent to the floor, push into your forearms to lift your torso. Slowly bring your knees closer together and take the Basic Child Pose (see page 288). Next, lie on your back and cross one thigh in front of the other, with both knees bent. Reach around to grasp your shins and rock slowly from side

2. If you don't feel you are sitting at six out of ten intensity and want to increase the challenge, you can take one forearm across the mat, while straightening the other arm forward. Rest your forehead on the forearm of the bent arm. If possible, reach both arms straight out in front, allowing your chest to touch the floor. If your neck feels healthy and up to the challenge over this long hold, have your chin on the floor, so that you look forward. Otherwise, place your forehead to the floor, as shown.

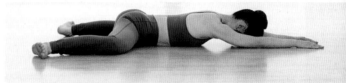

3. If you have gone beyond that first edge of six out of ten, then the options given above are too strong for your body. Try out Half-Frog: lengthen your left arm and leg out in one straight line, bend your right elbow and take it out wide, level with your right shoulder. Position your right knee out level with your hip, ankle flexed. Stay for three minutes, before coming out to work the second side.

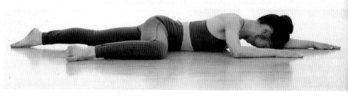

YIN FROG

to side. Change legs and rock again. Then spread out flat, with your arms and legs wide like a snow angel, for a minute or longer, to bask in the after-effects of your good efforts. This will allow the *chi* energy to circulate.

modifications and cautions

Use padding under your knees to protect them. Bringing your big toes together (called Tadpole Pose) will give much more comfort. Take more weight through the arms, as needed. Taking the arms wider apart brings more comfort in the shoulders. Long holds in this pose may not suit post-natal women. Before practising this pose, read the "Guidelines to your yin practice" on page 309.

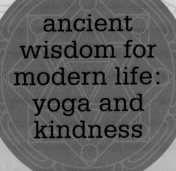

ancient wisdom for modern life: yoga and kindness

All of us, simply by virtue of being alive, act. This means that we all have the possibility to actively participate in the spiritual discipline of karma yoga – the yoga of action. Karma yoga is when you perform selfless acts of service, with no attachment to the outcome. Your actions, however simple or complex, are done

with a pure intent and your best efforts. Being detached from the outcome of your efforts acts to purify you of the usual cravings or aversions associated with the human experience. Caring for children, supporting a sick friend or simply doing your job to the best of your ability become spiritual markers if you approach them with a meditative mindset. Your actions become uplifting reminders that the universe is unfolding within you and through you. So important is karma

> *"Karma yoga is when you perform selfless acts of service, with no attachment to the outcome. Your actions, however simple or complex, are done with a pure intent and your best efforts."*

yoga that it is considered a path to Self-realization in its own right.

Altruism is a form of karma yoga. Studies have shown it to activate the subgenual cortex in the brain, and this is related to social attachment and bonding, in some species. Studies of volunteering – a form of altruism and karma yoga – show that we stay healthier and even live longer when we volunteer. It appears that altruism may be part of our neural wiring, in that we find it intrinsically pleasurable to help others, and doing so promotes social attachment and bonding. This mechanism actually seems to work both ways – altruistic acts promote happiness, and those who are happy are more likely to be kind.

Yoga philosophy tells us there will always be suffering around us. When you act to help others, don't try to fix anything. It will be more sustainable over the long term to let go of the outcome and simply offer your kindness.

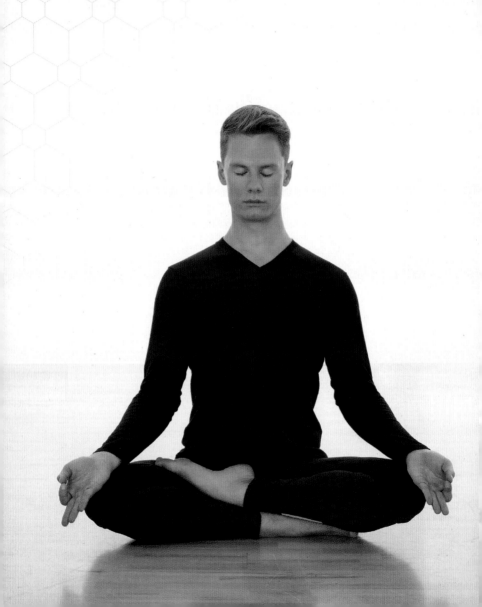

16

YOGA BREATH

Perhaps you have heard someone say, "If you can breathe, you can do yoga." This is often said as reassurance to someone with a stiff, aged or sore body, who – for whatever reason – is not able to attempt the more challenging postures. But the thing is: it's true. The breath connects us to the state of yoga. It brings us back to the *now* moment, the elusive state of existing in the present.

The breath opens us to life force. And sometimes yoga breathing feels like an insurance policy. For those times when you just don't feel like rolling out your mat. For those dark days when you feel too raw or wounded to launch into a sunny Sun Salute. On those dark nights that you may pass in deep grief. For those times when you can't get off to sleep. For those periods when you are too ill to move around much. You can, indeed, still practise yoga at these times. You can breathe and it can be supremely nourishing. And for the times when you feel good, happy and relaxed, too, yoga breathing will build your account balance of good energy for the future. What a miracle opening to your breathing can be. At any phase and at any time in your life, yoga breathing is relaxing, enjoyable and meditative.

the expansive breath

I appreciate this practice because every time I do it, I gather more information about how I breathe. I love the idea that like every snowflake, each breath is unique. This fills me with awe and helps me maintain a sense of wonder at each magical breath. So enjoy practising this often. Let it spark in you the curiosity of a child.

1. Settle yourself in any comfortable seated position. Rest one palm on your chest and take the back of the other hand to your mid-back area. Once your hands are in position, relax your shoulders as much as possible.

2. Close your eyes. Notice how your body moves to accommodate the breath. Let the light pressure of your hands enable you to notice how each inhalation expands you. Then allow the natural narrowing of the body to occur on each exhalation, and observe how both hands subtly descend.

3. After one to three minutes, slide the hands down, so that one is on your abdomen and the other on your lower back. Continue to watch each breath. Notice the relaxed blossoming outward of the belly as you inhale. Embrace the soft belly-breathing that comes with this full yogic breath. Observe the movements of the back. The changes here are subtle, so feel free to gently exaggerate your breathing, to better clarify how the lower back moves. Imagine the breath swirling around your lower back, dissolving any tension it meets. Stay here for one to three minutes.

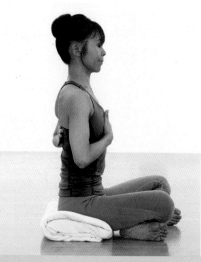

effects
Calming, focusing, revitalizing, nourishing

position
Choose any comfortable seated position where your spine is effortlessly upright. Pictured is the Happy Pose, also known as the Easy Cross-Legged Pose, where the seat is lifted by a folded blanket. Lifting your hips above your knees will free up your abdominal muscles to move more freely with the breath.

4. Change your arm position to wrap your palms around your side ribs, so that each set of fingers reaches toward the other. Check that you are cupping your ribcage rather than the waist, and that you can then soften the shoulders. If this position doesn't work well for you, cross your arms in front, to give yourself a hug, and wrap your palms around the sides of the ribcage. Notice how the breath moves into the sides of the torso. It's often helpful to consciously expand the intakes of air, to let the breath open into the side body. Notice how each inhalation will lift and broaden the ribs, while on each exhalation they drop down and narrow. Once you have done several slow, deeper-than-normal breaths, you may be able to return to a lighter breath and still sense this action of the ribs. Continue to practise for one to three minutes.

5. Now rest your hands on your thighs and continue to allow the torso to open on each inhalation and to condense on each exhalation. Let the breath feel full and wide. You may still feel the warm touch of the palms, as a reminder of where to breathe into. Visualize a balloon in the centre of the torso. Let it expand as you breathe in, and shrink a little as you breathe out. Imagine it expanding fairly uniformly in all directions – forward, backward and to each side. As you inhale, let it also expand downward toward the pelvic floor and upward toward the base of the throat. As you exhale, allow it to condense evenly, too. After one to three minutes of this calm breathing, prepare to come out slowly. Notice your degree of relaxation and how the ambience of the mind has changed.

take care
When you exaggerate the breathing to take in deeper breaths, keep it slow, rather than speeding it up. In particular, ensure the exhalations remain manageably slow.

☆ ocean breath

While I don't believe there is any one-size-fits-all practice in yoga, this Ocean Breath could be as close as it gets. Incorporating this into your yoga practice will give it a whole new sense of focus and flow. It allows you to tap into the majestic tidal ebb and flow of each sweeping, flowing breath.

This breath can be used as a standalone practice, but it can also be used throughout the entire active part of your physical yoga practice. It can take a short while to feel really comfortable with this breath, but it may take many months of regular practice to incorporate it fully into your yoga poses. However, it's so worth it. Integrating the Ocean Breath will elevate your whole physical yoga practice and give it that sense of moving meditation that we often long for – and then you will understand why its Sanskrit name, *ujjayi*, is translated as "victorious breath".

1. The exhalation part of this Ocean Breath is the easiest part to pick up first. Bring a small constriction to the airway at the base of the throat, and breathe out slowly through an open mouth. As you do this, make a sigh, like you're fogging up a mirror. You will make a light throaty noise, like the sound of a snoring baby. Notice how your throat feels warm. As you relax into this part of the practice, your exhalation may start to lengthen out. Be sure to allow your inhalations to extend correspondingly, in order to stay balanced.

2. Move from the open-mouthed exhalation to the closed mouth. Keep that same throaty breath, but place your lips together and send the air out though the nostrils. You'll experience the air moving through the throat, and it almost feels as if the nostrils are bypassed. The sound will be a little smaller, but still audible to anyone right next to you. After a minute or so, take a rest. If you feel comfortable, continue to the next stage. If it feels stressful, stop for now and practice for short lengths of time over days and weeks, until it feels easy.

YOGA BREATH

effects
Focusing, warming, meditative, grounding, restful

position
Lie down or sit in any comfortable upright position. Pictured is Perfect Pose, a wide cross-legged posture, with one ankle on top of the other and the feet snuggled in close to the body, to tuck in the toes. Use this throughout your Hatha yoga practice while you hold each posture and when transitioning mindfully between poses.

3. Still constricting the airway, inhale. It can be helpful to imagine that you're breathing through a little hole at the base of the throat. Check that the breath really does feel as if it comes from the throat, and that it's not a nasal sound. Although there is a constriction at the throat, you need to feel softness and ease there. Work on getting a constant rate of air flow on both parts of the breath – in and out. Both inhalation and exhalation should have a sound like the distant ocean. Enjoy the tidal flow of your breath. Practise this glottal breathing for anywhere from a minute up to the full duration of your yoga practice, breaking from it during your final relaxation to return to your natural breath.

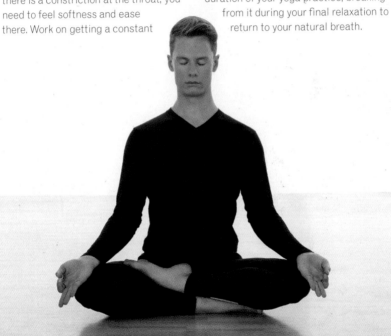

take care
Yoga breathwork is a personal thing and varies from person to person. If you feel something isn't suiting you on any level – physically, mentally or emotionally – do consult an experienced yoga teacher. Discontinue if you feel light-headed or dizzy.

rectangular breath

It's hard to beat this, as a wonderfully energizing practice, and I often start my classes with some version or other of it. I love the way it makes the lungs feel light and expanded. Each breath is slowed and allowed to expand out into its four parts.

There is dedicated time for the two retentions: the nourishing fullness of the inhalation and that delightful emptiness of the exhalation. The pause after the inhalation allows you to get the most energy from that intake of air. Both pauses deepen your concentration, as does the mental counting. Counting takes the mind away from those mundane everyday thoughts and moves it into that elusive present-moment awareness, which elevates us and makes us feel happy. I hope you fall in love with this exercise, too.

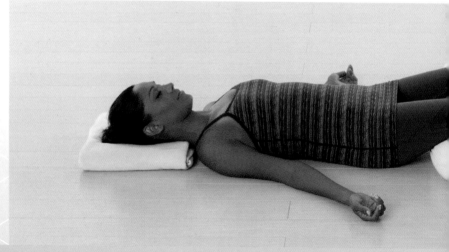

effects

Revitalizing, expanding, energy-enhancing, focusing, quietening

position

Sit comfortably or lie down. What's great about lying down is that all those muscles that usually hold you up don't need to work as hard, because the body is fully supported by the earth. So any muscles that have dual breathing and postural roles can now dedicate themselves to their task of supporting a full, deep breath.

1. Sit comfortably tall or, better still, lie down. Begin with a clean slate, by letting the air flow out of your lungs. Now inhale while you take a slow count of four. Maintain a steady rate of air flow through the nostrils. Rather than starting with a stronger or faster initial inhalation, which ends with a strangled flow, this is more controlled. Meter the timing, so that this constant air flow fills the lungs to comfortably brimming, just as you reach the number four.

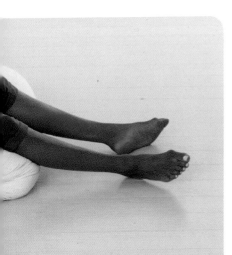

2. Now invite the breath to linger, as you would invite a much-loved guest to linger in your home. Hold the breath in for two counts. Enjoy the way your ribcage has opened to allow you to hold this full breath. Check that your facial muscles and tissues are soft. Release any unnecessary hardness or holding in your body.

3. Exhale during a count of four. As with the inhalation part of the breath, aim to maintain a constant rate of air flow from the nostrils, timing it so that you are empty as you reach four.

4. Hold your breath out for two beats. Sink into the soothing quiet that comes with this emptiness. Like floating effortlessly on top of a still pond, it's a chance to really touch that nugget of stillness that resides within us always, but which can easily be lost in a busy modern life.

5. You have now completed one round. Start your next four-beat inhalation and continue on for another five to 15 rounds. Then relax all efforts and rest while you absorb the benefits of the practice.

take care
Don't hold the breath in if you have high blood pressure. Avoid holding the breath in or out during pregnancy.

modification
If the 4:2:4:2 ratio of inhale: pause: exhale: pause feels manageable, step it up by lengthening the active parts of the breath. Breathe in and out for a count of five, while maintaining the two-beat pauses. If this 5:2:5:2 ratio works well for you, increase it again to 6:3:6:3, so that you are breathing in and out for six counts, and holding the breath for three.

RECTANGULAR BREATH

golden-thread breathing

This is a terrific anti-anxiety breathing practice, which allows you to take a step back from any of your cares and worries. You will practise being a passive observer, not needing to react against or interact with any issues or concerns. It reminds me that I am pure, perfect and complete just as I am. We realize there is actually no need to change anything at all in order to experience wholeness and serenity.

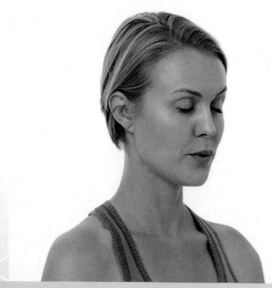

effects

Calming, soothing, healing

position

It's best to be upright for this practice. Kneeling postures, cross-legged options or seated on a chair are all suitable. If you are cross-legged on the floor, it's helpful to have some support under your seat. Anatomically, when the hips are lifted in comparison to the knees, it will be easier to draw yourself up tall, to maintain the full dignity of your posture.

1. Sit comfortably with your eyes closed and notice the rate and depth of your respiration. Breathing through your nose, spend some time noticing how long your inhalations are. Then move your mind to your exhalations and observe how long they are.

2. Continue to inhale through your nostrils, but move the exhalation to your mouth. Let your lips be wide and soft, and allow the air to flow out soundlessly. If it feels comfortable and effortless, narrow the distance between the lips – perhaps bringing them so close together as to imagine holding a paper tissue between them. This narrow aperture should create no tension around your soft lips. It should assist the exhalation in lengthening out a little, so do ensure that you keep a nicely balanced breath. Continue to take leisurely inhalations though both nostrils.

3. Each time you exhale, feel the touch of the air leaving the body and visualize it as a fine golden thread of air extending out in front of you. As the exhalations are slow and unhurried, your slender golden thread may undulate softly. As the exhalations are long, so the thread extends out, perhaps surprisingly far.

4. At the end of this golden thread, place any worries or concerns that you have. I like to imagine a neat little cane basket floating out in front, ready to accept anything I want to put in it. Without speeding up the breathing at all, continue to watch this basket. The beautiful thing about observing these concerns is that they are now externalized. Being out in front, they are no longer a part of you. You can experience yourself freely, without these troubles.

5. To close, decide where you would like to place the issues at the end of your golden thread. It's up to your imagination, so it can be anywhere at all. And it's also up to you whether or not you choose to take any of them back. Then return to your easy breathing, in and out through the nose, to calmly watch the breath for several minutes.

take care
Do seek advice from a professional if you need further help.

modification
If practising with the eyes closed takes you to dark places that you don't want to visit, then open your eyes.

tibetan alternate-nostril breathing

Alternate-nostril breathing, or *Nadi Shodhana*, is traditionally done to harmonize the right-and left-brain hemispheres and purify the energy meridians. If this sounds like fanciful yogic folklore to you, keep in mind that yoga practitioners the world over swear by this one and love the effects. This take on the classic alternate-nostril breathing is a super practice, day or night, which adds quality to your life. It is great in the morning, to set you up for a calm and more focused day; beneficial at night, to decompress after a long day or help you go off to sleep; fabulous before or after a meeting; and lovely to lead you into meditation. Try it out and claim your bit of bliss!

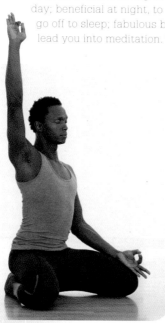

1. Sit in a comfortable upright position. Place a hand on each thigh, palm up and the tips of your thumbs and index fingers touching. Take your right arm out to the side and, as you inhale, sweep it in a wide arc to bring it overhead. Do this over a count of five beats. The wide arm sweeps encourage slightly longer inhalations, which means that the exhalations will also tend to elongate and the whole system can settle.

effects

Calming, harmonizing, balancing, focusing

position

Choose your most comfortable position. Pictured is a wide-kneed Hero Pose, but any posture that allows you to sit upright without excess effort is fine. You may prefer a supported kneeling option, or cross-legged with your seat on a cushion. If using a chair, resist leaning into the chair back, but sit tall using your own muscle power.

YOGA BREATH

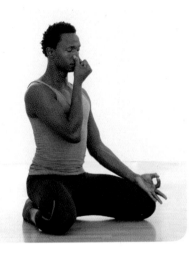 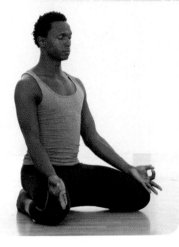

2. Once the arm is overhead, hold your breath in for a count of three while you bend your right elbow to lower your arm. Use your right thumb to cover your right nostril. With your right nostril now closed, exhale out of your left nostril for a count of eight beats. Once your lungs have emptied, hold the breath out for three counts while you lower your right hand to rest on your thigh again.

3. Now change the arms so that you raise your left arm for five beats. Hold in your breath for three, as you lower your arm and cover your left nostril. Breathe out through your right nostril for a count of eight. Hold the empty breath for three, as you lower your left hand to rest on the thigh. This is one complete round. Continue, alternating right and left arms, for five to ten more rounds, finishing with the exhale through the right nostril. Then sit quietly and absorb the way the textures of the mind have changed.

take care

It's completely normal to have one nostril slightly more open than the other. If one nostril feels blocked to the point of discomfort, try only partially covering the other nostril, so that the restricted side can still maximize the flow of air as much as is doable.

modification

Feel free to count off the beats slower or faster, if you wish to. Ensure the 5:3:8:3 ratio works for you. Talk to an experienced yoga teacher if you think you'd prefer a different ratio – there are lots of other options.

ancient wisdom for modern life: the causes of suffering

PARINAMA TAPA
SAMSKARADUKHAIH
GUNAVRITTIVIRODHACCA
DUKHAMEVA SARVAM
VIVEKINAHH

परिणामतापसस्कारदुःखैर्गुणवृत्तिविरोधा
च्च दुःखमेव सर्वं विवेकिन

Yoga Sutras II:15

This *sutra* speaks of the causes of suffering, and the first cause on the list is change, *parinama*. All matter is subject to change. As no matter is constant, change is inevitable, yet it disturbs us. The suffering around change can come from four sources:

- Suffering is created when things change around you that impact on what you feel in a negative way. For example, you lose your job or something special to you.
- We also suffer from what we don't have, but want. There are cravings both small and large. Not getting that promotion, not finding your "one true love", a delay in receiving your morning coffee, any

"Change can be a cause of suffering. All matter is subject to change. As no matter is constant, change is inevitable, yet it disturbs us."

time you find yourself wishing for more of an experience that you found pleasurable in the past.

• A third cause of suffering is conditioning from the past, *samskaras* (see page 356). This is when you repeat patterns or behaviour, consciously or unconsciously, which don't serve you or are even harmful.

• Finally, changes within yourself – at least undesirable changes – will also cause suffering.

> *"The effects of the gunas can be seen in the seasons, the food we eat, the lifestyle we choose. The gunas act on our thoughts, our desires, our moods and our personalities."*

WHAT CAUSES CHANGE?

A key concept in Indian philosophy is that of the *gunas*. The word *guna* means "string" or "strand", and these threads weave together to form all of creation, past and present. There are three *gunas*, and they are important to understand because the origin of change is simply the fluctuation of these *gunas*.

The three *gunas* are *rajas*, *tapas* and *sattva*. *Rajas* is the energy of creation, motion, passion, action and preservation. *Tamas*, its opposite, is the energy of destruction, inertia, heaviness and disorder. *Sattva* contains the qualities of peace, harmony, wholesomeness, lucidity and balance. Each of these *gunas* is present in us and in every single thing around us. They don't act like a simple

THE THREE *GUNAS*:

RAJAS
The energy of creation, motion, passion, action and preservation.

TAMAS
The energy of destruction, inertia, heaviness and disorder.

SATTVA
Peace, harmony, wholesomeness, lucidity and balance.

"on" or "off" switch. Instead, while the *gunas* are always present, they fluctuate in relative dominance. These fluctuations are what create change and the rate of change. Their state of flux may be fast or incredibly slow. Your bad mood can change the instant you receive terrific news. Conversely, while the enormous oceans appear to remain constant, science tells us they are changing, too.

The presence of the *gunas* can be observed acting on us all the time: they give the various flavours to the different times of day as we switch between work, rest and play. The effects of the *gunas* can be seen in the seasons, the food we eat and the lifestyle we choose. The *gunas* act on our thoughts, our desires, our moods and our personalities.

HOW CAN I DEAL WITH CHANGE?

We understand that all matter (including our own matter), being subject to the *gunas*, will change. It's inevitable. We also understand from the yoga teachings that no one can avoid suffering. Even the most enlightened yogis will experience the effects of change, simply because they still have a body.

Knowing that change is affected by the relative dominance and balance of the differing qualities of the *gunas* is actually very empowering, as we can consciously choose to take action to redress any imbalance. We can decrease or increase any of the qualities, usually by doing something in the opposite direction. Often the simplest of things will balance you out. For instance, you can counter feeling tired and heavy by a light and energetic activity, such as dancing or a flowing yoga practice. On the other hand, if you need to sleep but find your mind is still on active alert, ensuring that your room is dark, eliminating screen-time and drinking a liquid such as milk, which has a heavy energy, will support the quality of inertia that is required for sleep.

Change is a problem for us when our thoughts and feelings are habitual, rather than adaptive, and have trouble shifting to accept the change. It can take time for our nervous system to assimilate change. And if our chronic stress response is reinforced during this process, it can feel really hard even to access our capacity for change. The stress created by change can lead to anxiety or depression. When we can choose to *respond* to our experience, rather than react, we create the optimal conditions to assimilate change.

Awareness can support us in recognizing any resistance to change that we may be experiencing and examine it more closely. Rather than pushing away or collapsing in the face of change, we can become curious about what exactly is happening at a deeper level, and hold ourselves with great kindness as we potentially explore new ways of being.

It may sound bleak, but it's not. Change is also an empowering tool – you can change your mind at any time. Understanding how inevitable change is can shift you from victim mode (poor me, why me?), because the reality is actually "why *not* me?" It can help you to move on from unhelpful emotions like blame, guilt and regret. It's possible to influence change in a positive direction. The experience of suffering will provide the energy to search for a solution.

Understanding that we are all subject to suffering, and that someone else's pain could be your own, allows you to cultivate compassion. We know there is no hierarchy of suffering. No one person's difficulties are any less legitimate than another's. Keep in mind that even the same painful event will be experienced with different intensities by different individuals. Practise the Loving-Kindness Meditation (see page 372) and the Gratitude Meditation (see page 370).

Awareness and self-enquiry are stepping stones to dealing with suffering. Yoga practices, and particularly meditation, can help in clarifying your perception and keeping you connected to that serene, greater Self (practise the Mindfulness Meditation on page 366). This will mean that you can meet those inevitable shifts, heartbreaks, yearnings or painful patterns with equanimity and then move forward with grace.

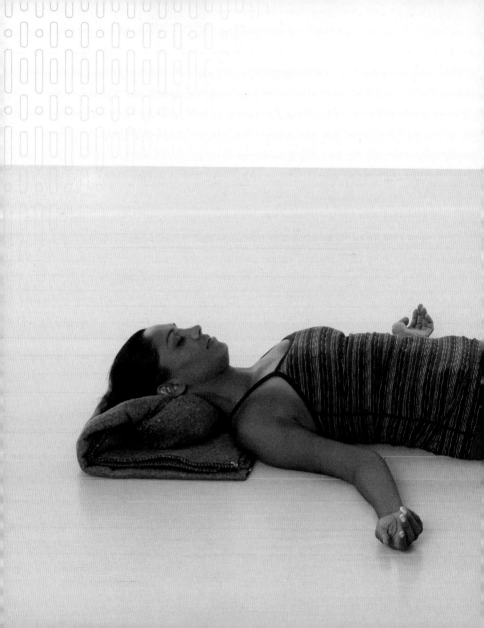

17

RELAXATIONS
TO REVEL IN

For many people, their smartphone is the first thing they touch in the morning and the last thing they check at night. Busyness has crowded out spaciousness. Spaciousness is the opposite of stress and a key factor in relieving it. Where stress makes you feel contracted and tight, spaciousness is loose and expansive. The bottom line is: spaciousness feels *goooood.*

Yoga postures enable the body to feel spacious inside. They help counter stress simply through the mind–body connection. That feels good. But what feels even better is to close every practice that you do with a relaxation, like the ones that follow.

Stay resting in one of these reclining postures as long as you can. It takes about 15 minutes for the physical body to relax. Your bones will feel heavy and your muscles can release. Your mind will start to slow, and you'll drift through various stages of release. While you may still notice your thoughts, there will be less identification with them. You can

sometimes drop into an even deeper state, where you are awake and yet disconnected from the outer world. It's a special space you don't know you have entered until you come back from it. And, like your thoughts, any noises just wash over you, leaving you undisturbed.

I'll tell you a secret. Even if you have had no time, been too tired, or for any other reason have not done a single yoga posture, you can *still* do a beautiful life-enhancing relaxation. If you need to justify why you are taking 20 minutes' time-out, tell yourself that the more switched on you have become, the more time-efficiently you need to learn to switch off. And, with practice, you will become more efficient at relaxation.

But I hope you don't feel the need to justify taking this time, because you deserve to recharge. You deserve to feel the world drop away as you detach from your thoughts. You deserve to experience the delightful qualities of spaciousness and emptiness. Because it feels good. And to feel good is your birthright.

serenity relaxation

Supremely relaxing, this gentle, comforting practice will open your heart and soothe your mind. The world needs more gentleness and kindness. Imagine this practice healing not only yourself, but also all others who need it.

set-up suggestion: corpse pose with neck roll

Lie on your back with a folded blanket under your head. Create a small roll to support the curve of the neck. Check that your forehead is slightly higher than your chin. Make any fine adjustments to ensure that you feel comfortable enough to commit to stillness. Just as when you throw a pebble into a still pond it disturbs the water, so any movements made while in deep relaxation will send ripples of disturbance though your system. If you are pregnant, use a bolster lengthways under your spine, or lie on your left side and place one pillow under your head and another between your thighs.

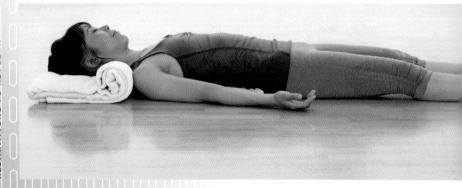

1. Choose your favourite resting position. Have your arms out to the sides, with palms facing up. Take time to check your level of comfort and cushioning and to release any last fidgets. Take your awareness to your hands. With the palms soft and fingers gently curled in relaxation, imagine you are breathing in and out of your palms. Each time you inhale, imagine both palms absorbing the air; and each time you exhale, experience your breath flowing out of the palms. Stay with this for a minute or two. You may observe that this simple act of watching your breath will help it to slow down, which enhances the relaxation effect.

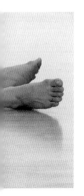

2. Do the same with your feet. With each inhalation, sense your breath moving into your body through the soles of your feet. Then, without any hurry at all, allow the air to exit through the feet as well. Experience your feet becoming open and transparent as you enjoy the process over the next one to two minutes.

3. Next, move your awareness to your abdomen. Again, as if you didn't need your lungs to breathe, visualize the air moving in through your navel, and exhale out from your navel centre. Notice how your belly moves in response to each of the stages of your breath. Stay with this for a minute or two.

4. Now move your focus to your heart centre in the middle of your chest. Inhale, directing your breath in through this space, and experience yourself exhaling directly through it, too. Repeat this for one minute. Then start to inhale *calm* through your heart centre. Allow your heart to fill up with this calm, and each time you exhale, let it diffuse out through your whole body. Enjoy the process of collecting it as you inhale, and then leisurely letting it go, to filter out in all directions – through your torso, along your limbs to the tips of your fingers and toes, and releasing gently into the head.

5. After a minute or two, change your focus word. Inhale *kindness* into your heart. Enjoy your naturally lengthened exhalations and, each time you breathe in, simply inhale kindness. Enjoy the release that naturally occurs each time you breathe out, and start to spread that through the body. Enjoy receiving the energy that comes with each inhalation of kindness, then letting it go as it spreads over the shoulders and down the arms to the hands. Let it spread over the hips on its way down the legs to the toes. Let kindness diffuse up into the head. Stay with this for two minutes, or as long as you wish, then let go of all efforts and float for a while. Come out slowly with a soft smile.

☆ energy-balancing relaxation

This practice is ingenious. It works whichever end of the spectrum you find yourself at. Whether your mind starts off fatigued, heavy and dull, or whether your thought patterns are speedy, scattered and darting, this relaxation will help re-centre and re-balance you. The clever use of directional breathing will bring you closer to the nugget of calm that always resides within you.

set-up suggestion: corpse pose with weighted palms

Lie on your back, with your hands beside your hips and your feet comfortably wide. Try taking your arms a little wider than they might be initially and allow the shoulders to soften. Likewise, take your feet one notch wider than you might already have them, and sense whether that could enable you to relax more easily. The body often likes a little weight on it, so try placing a light weight such as an eye-pillow on each palm, with your thumbs draped on top. Place another eye-pillow over the heart centre. Cover the eyes with a fourth eye-pillow. If you are pregnant, use a bolster lengthways under your spine, or lie on your left side and place one pillow under your head and another between your thighs.

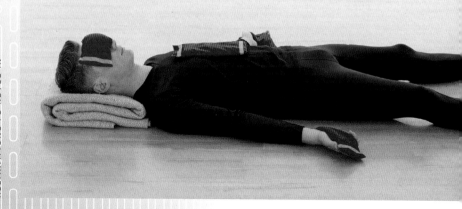

1. Choose your preferred relaxation position. Take your focus to the exhalation part of each breath. Each time you breathe out, exhale down from the crown of the head, through the throat to the heart centre in the middle of the chest. Stay with this

for a minute or more. Your only task is to track that exhalation downward. Appreciate the sense of happy unravelling as you let go with each exhalation. Each exhale takes you closer to stillness and silence. Enjoy that.

2. Next, add the inhalations to your awareness. Direct each inhalation upward, so that each one starts at the navel and travels up to the heart centre. You now have a focal point for each part of the breath. On each full yogic breath, you will inhale and follow the breath up from the navel to the heart. On each exhalation, you'll drop your awareness from the crown of the

head down to the heart. Continue this process for two or three minutes.

3. While you are running the energies up and down your body, you are helping to balance out the dualities within. The opposite forces of heaviness and lightness come better into balance. Areas of deficiency and excess can even out. You will feel expansive and yet grounded, playful and yet determined, and will balance silence with action. Masculine and feminine, and any other opposite qualities residing within you, will become less distant. You'll be able to experience how being in balance is so much more comfortable than being out of balance.

4. Give a colour to each of part of the breath. Perhaps black for the rising breath, and white for the falling breath. Over the next few breaths, visualize these two colours meeting at the heart. Allow them to twirl into a flowing spiral. Breathe into this spiral of colour, allowing it to swell, then as you exhale let the colours diffuse through the whole body. Continue this for another minute or, if you have time, longer. Then just stay resting for a while. When you are ready to come out, sense your physical body. Make tiny movements with your fingers and toes. Expand those movements to your ankles and wrists. Move and stretch in any way that feels good. Open the eyes and return slowly and gracefully to your outer world.

☆ peaceful mind relaxation

This relaxation is about the quickest and easiest way I know for everyone from beginners to experienced yogis to flick that switch from stress to serenity. It's such a good way to declutter the mind that I've even been known to practise it over about 12 breaths in the supermarket queue. Taking 20 minutes to lie down in a quiet space is even better.

set-up suggestion: corpse pose with neck support

Shown here is the Corpse Pose, *Savasana*, with the natural curve of the neck supported by a roll created from a folded blanket. Check the height of your blanket roll, so that your forehead is slightly higher than your chin. In addition to the neck roll, tuck the blanket under at the side corners, to cradle the sides of your head as a winged aeroplane seat does.

When your head is completely supported in this symmetrical position, your neck muscles will no longer need to work subtly, to hold your head steady, and you will relax more easily. If you are pregnant, use a bolster lengthways under your spine, or lie on your left side and place one pillow under your head and another between your thighs.

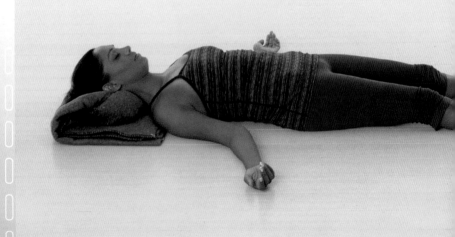

1. Choose your most comfortable relaxation position, taking time to fine-tune any props and positioning yourself so that you don't cheat yourself out of feeling supremely comfortable. With your eyes closed, check in with your breath. As you breathe in, simply think of your head. Then, when you breathe out, think of your chest. For the next ten or so breaths, continue moving between these two areas of focus: head to chest. This is the beginning of the process of getting excess energy out of the head, by drawing it lower down in the body.

2. Next, each time you inhale, take the breath into your chest. When you exhale, think of your lower-back area. Allow yourself to breathe out of your lower back, letting it soften and lengthen. Notice the completely unforced, natural expansion of your upper torso as you take each breath in through the front of the chest. When you breathe out through the lower back and kidney area, allow any lower-back tensions to dissipate. Let any hardness in the lower back dissolve. Continue this chest/lower-back focus for ten breaths or longer.

3. Finally, lower your focus to move it between your lower back and your feet. Take your inhalations into your lower back. Enjoy the expansion in your lower back as it absorbs your breath. Breathe out though the soles of your feet. Let your lower back and kidneys soak up the breath in an unhurried way, and drop your energy down to your feet as they let go of each exhalation. Continue this practice for ten breaths or longer. Then notice any differences in the textures of your mind compared to when you started.

☆ floating relaxation

This practice is brilliant to settle a busy mind, and a great help
to calm you off to sleep. You will also understand how coming
home to yourself is infinitely nourishing.

set-up suggestion: with cushioned head, knees, ankles and wrists

If you have six or seven blankets, try out this
position. To form a support for the backs of
the knees, use either a yoga bolster or two
blankets, folded three times and then rolled
up together, Roll up a single blanket to place
under your Achilles – the ankle arch just above
your heel bone. It should be half the height
of the knee roll. Fold another blanket to make
a pillow for your head. Test out the height –
when you lie back, your forehead should be level
with, or slightly higher than, your chin. Use one
more blanket to lift each forearm slightly. Ensure
that you will be warm, so cover yourself with
another blanket if necessary. If you are pregnant,
use a bolster lengthways under your spine, or lie
on your left side and place one pillow under your
head and another between your thighs.

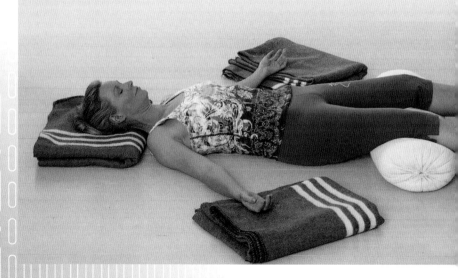

1. Choose your most comfortable lying position. Scan over your body to check that you feel luxuriously comfortable. If anything needs adjusting, take the time to do so.

Sometimes the mind can latch onto the smallest of discomforts or asymmetries, and this will impede your journey into deep relaxation.

2. Notice the expansive qualities of every inhalation. Observe how each one gently fills your belly and chest. In classic relaxed yogic breathing, the belly will move first, followed by the chest, as the air is drawn into the lungs. But don't try too hard. Simply allow whatever is there to be there. Each inhalation will subtly lift you. Open yourself to a sense of floating every time you breathe in.

3. After a few minutes, begin to notice the releasing qualities of each exhalation. Allow each exhalation to float you down, as if you get a little heavier as you breathe out. This sinking effect can feel like coming home. Come home to your true essential nature. Peaceful you. Pure you. Calm you. Content you. Joyful you. Blissful you. Let all the other noise of life drop away as you continue to follow your breath, floating with each inhalation and sinking with each exhalation. Stay like this for another few minutes.

4. Now start to count your breathing backward from 33 down to one. Mentally repeat your yourself: "I am breathing in 33, I am breathing out 33; I am breathing in 32, I am breathing out 32," and so on down to one. If you lose track, return to 33 and start again. The purpose is not necessarily to reach one, but simply to count yourself into a deeply restful space. If you reach one, release all efforts. Just float.

5. When it's time to come back, feel the touch of the floor and supports underneath you, as if you have just floated on warm tropical waters and arrived at the sandy shore. Let the sandy bed come up underneath your body. Experience how good it feels in your physical body to be this relaxed. Check in with the atmosphere of your mental body. Notice the textures of your emotional body. If you believe in a fourth dimension, check in with your soul body, too. With all these dimensions harmoniously wrapped up in your physical body, you will be ready to resume your day, revitalized and alive.

FLOATING RELAXATION

ancient wisdom for modern life

SAMSKARAS संस्कार

A *samskara* is a psychological imprint that causes us to repeat patterns of behaviour. Yoga philosophy teaches us that every action we take and every intention we have will create an impression, a *samskara*. *Samskaras* show up in our tendencies and habits, and become part of our character structure.

Each *samskara* was originally of value in our lives and provides us with pleasure or allows us to avoid suffering. However, any *samskara* – even that which originally created pleasure – has the potential to create suffering, as the purpose it serves in our lives changes as our lives alter. Suffering will be created if we don't change the patterns in our lives to respond to our life changes. Suffering is created when our lived experience of the present doesn't match our previous experience (or our projected idea of what our current experience "should" be). In other words, suffering is caused by our inability to accept that everything – including ourselves – is subject to change, and that change is constant.

Samskaras rule our lives in ways we don't even notice. These habits and unconscious patterns cause us to react in ways that may no longer be helpful. Rather than consciously responding to life as it currently is, the first step in dealing with *samskaras* is awareness, so that we can know exactly who is driving the bus we are on. Under the yoga precept of self-study – *svadhyaya* – you can develop the self-awareness to determine what it is about your behaviour that you want to change, and can analyse what is holding this behaviour in place. It can be helpful to consider the *gunas* here (see page 342). If *tamas* is dominant, it is likely to manifest in feelings of heaviness, inertia, laziness, procrastination and feeling "stuck". A predominance of *rajas* may feel rewarding initially, as you can get lots done, but you may be over-stimulated by the continual On-switch into the passion, action and excitement this *guna* generates. A shortage of *sattva* shows up as not having the clarity of mind to clearly perceive the situation that you are facing and to plan the steps or tasks ahead.

HOW TO ERADICATE THE *SAMSKARAS*

Consider the results of your *samskaras*. What are you getting out of the situation as it is? If you can reduce the attachment to the result, you will weaken the *samskara*. Each thought and action is a seed that will grow. It's important to cut the negative thought-seeds before they get to the threshold of creating a strong *samskara*, which is harder to root out. The more often you indulge a habitual pattern, the more you strengthen the neural pathways in the brain responsible for giving you a sense of satisfaction, pleasure or pain, and the harder it is to change. This is great when you are a classical musician and you practise diligently to perform at your best. But it's not so great if you practise indulging in sensual pleasures, such as over-eating, when you really would like to lose weight.

So root out *samskaras* early, and be diligent when you notice the patterns sneaking back in. Practising yoga on a regular basis gives you a constant reference point, so that you can keep track of your experience and continually refresh your internal "browser" and keep it up to date. Your yoga practice can support you to notice at a deeper level any habitual tendencies that

> *"Eradicate those thought patterns that can send you into a downward spiral. When you catch it occurring, tell yourself to stop it: remember that you are a powerful being!"*

are not in alignment with your chosen goals or values. Awareness is the key to change. Practising new behaviours in the direction that you consciously choose to follow will strengthen new neural pathways, and over time it will weaken any unconscious pathways that were the basis of known and familiar previous patterns of thought and behaviour.

Eradicate any "stinking thinking" – those thought patterns that can send you into a downward spiral. When you catch it occurring, tell yourself to stop it: remember that you are a powerful being. Becoming aware takes practice. Once you have spent some time creating a clearer mind, your thought patterns will become more obvious to you, and you

will become better at discriminating between thoughts that are beneficial to your well-being and thought-patterns that may lead to less optimal states of being.

Think about what you are planting with your thoughts, intents and feelings. What is it that you really want to grow? Replace unhelpful thoughts with a more appropriate and true thought-stream, which will create new neural pathways. Remember: with neuroplasticity, we know that neurons that fire together, wire together. If you starve the seed to weaken that *samskara* while you create and strengthen the positive, you are on your way. And do consult a professional if you need help analysing the causes or dealing with the effects of your *samskaras*.

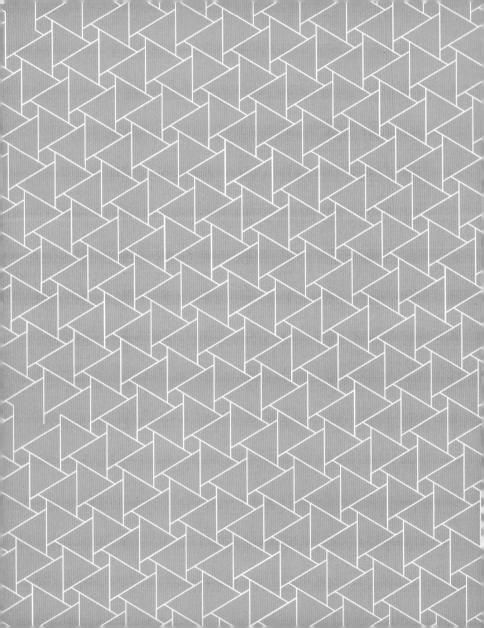

Part 4

YOGA MIND

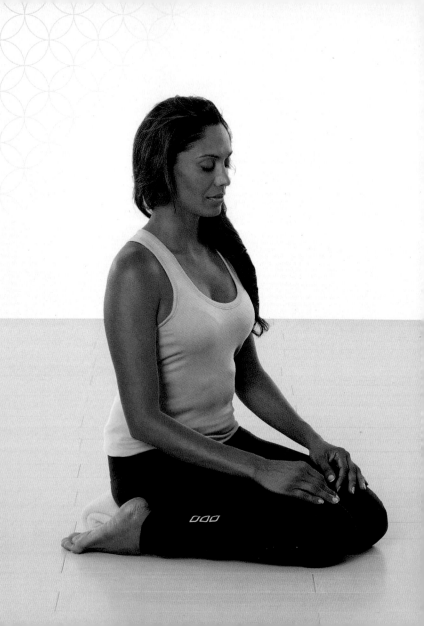

18.
IN THE MOOD: MEDITATIONS

Some people think meditation is a particular mood, like a goal to be reached. But meditation is not a mood. It's a quality of mind that can incorporate all moods. Other people despair of their busy minds, declaring, "I can't meditate." The thing is: it is the very nature of your mind to be busy and create thoughts. But you don't need to stop the thinking to benefit from meditation practice. Instead, create equanimity by disassociating yourself from distracting or disturbing thoughts. In this way, by changing your relationship with your thoughts, you can come out of suffering.

When we are able to let go of any frustrations, discomforts or sleepiness we meet on the path, we open to the calm, abiding effect of meditation. And then we find that meditation helps us to become more grounded and resilient, less reactive to triggers, and simply more content.

Disconnect to reconnect

We live in a fast and furiously efficient world. Technology has given us some freedoms, but it has bound us in other ways. It's now so easy to be constantly available for your job and to fall into work overload. Even our quiet time might involve staring at a screen, with a weekend spent binge-watching, Web-surfing or pinging and liking on social media. So it's more important than ever to disconnect from the sea of technology and connect back to ourselves. It's time to move on from wired-and-tired, and step up to be inspired.

We wear "busy" like a badge of honour. There is even a term for it: "Western laziness and Eastern laziness". Eastern laziness means not fully stepping up to life. After all, with the possibility of another incarnation, you could be tempted to take it easy, to the detriment of not realizing your full potential in this life. Western laziness, on the other hand, means not having the discipline or the ability to say no. There is so much encouragement to do more that we race around, as modern life seduces us outside ourselves.

What happens to us when we are stressed?

Stress means that many people are tuned in and switched on all the time, and have unlearned how to tune out and centre down. Stress seems to be the new norm. It's what we *expect* to feel. Under stress, our adrenaline-based nervous system kicks in. When we are under stress, we go on hyper-alert. It doesn't even matter whether or not the stress is real. Even the perception of stress will switch on our "fight or flight" mechanism.

With the release of stress hormones, blood supply is diverted away from the "not essential in an emergency" organs of the digestive and reproductive systems and is sent to the "this is an emergency, I might have to run away from the lion" parts of the body. Is it any wonder that so many people suffer from digestive problems and have trouble with infertility? Glucose levels rise, increasing the risk of diabetes; we find ourselves too wired to fall asleep, or wake up in the early hours and can't get back to sleep. Under stress, the blood vessels constrict and the heart beats faster, increasing the risk of high blood pressure, heart disease or a stroke. The immune system is suppressed, making us more susceptible to disease. We suffer from fatigue and exhaustion.

What's the good news?

Regular meditation or mindfulness practice has consistently been shown to reduce stress and stress-related illness. It switches off the "fight or flight" response, can lower blood pressure, supports the immune system and reduces stress-related illness, such as heart disease, depression and anxiety. Sleep quality, cognitive abilities, coping skills and interpersonal relationships are enhanced. The faster you live and the more stressful your life, the more important it is to find efficient mechanisms to decompress – and meditation might be exactly the antidote you need.

DISCONNECT TO RECONNECT

mindfulness meditation

Mindfulness meditation is a moment-to-moment non-judgemental awareness. It teaches us how to be present to life as it unfolds. As the external world is constantly feeding us with experiences, this practice allows us to use them to move

positioning idea

Shown is Lotus Pose, *Padmasana*, which is harder than it looks, so do warm up first. Try Perfect Pose if this is not comfortable for you. To fold in the right leg, bend your knee and allow the thigh to fall out to the right. Take hold of the foot and slide it on top of the left thigh, bringing the heel as close to the left hip as possible. Externally rotate your left thigh, allowing the knee and toes to fall to the left. Bend the knee to hold your foot and squeeze your right knee towards the floor. Carefully slide the left ankle on top of the right to bring the heel towards the hip. Place your hands in *Jnana mudra*, with the thumb and the index finger forming a circle.

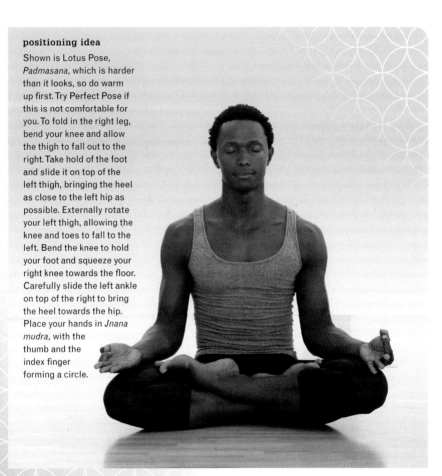

toward the higher goal of realization of the Self. Even if you are not quite aiming to get to that point, you'll still notice an abundance of benefits along the way. Mindfulness meditation is a beautiful antidote to the craziness of modern life.

1. Relax. Choose a comfortable upright position, such as Perfect Pose (page 332).

2. Breathe. Observe the rate and depth of your respiration. When observing the sensations of the breath, find the most obvious places for you. It might be movements of the chest or the belly. It could be the air moving through the nostrils, or the touch of the air on the skin of the upper lip. Use your chosen point to help draw in your focus. Each time you breathe in, you simply know that you are breathing in. Each time you breathe out, you just know you are breathing out.

3. Watch. Observe your stream of thoughts from the point of view of a passive witness. It's a bit like sitting by a highway and watching the cars pass. Obviously you are not the cars (your thoughts that arise are); you are a silent observer of the stream of thoughts. What may happen as you sit by the highway is that you find you have boarded the bus of your thoughts and it's taken you off on a trip somewhere else. Meditation is simply about beginning again. Wake up

to the awareness that you have lost your witnessing self by jumping on that bus, and hop off it. So much of meditation practice is really about remembering to come back. And as it will happen over and over again, smile kindly on yourself and simply begin again. Remember: any upset will only send ripples of disturbance through your system, which is counterproductive.

4. Allow. Let your experience be what it is. Mindfulness is a non-dual practice. No one thing is considered more special than another. Nothing is omitted from mindfulness practice. Everything in your field of awareness is cherished, just because it's in your field. There is no pushing away the "bad" or craving the "good". Continue to observe your thoughts with a gentle curiosity. Awareness is non-invasive. Awareness doesn't alter what we are noticing, so there are no biases. It is also illuminative. It shines a light on what is, right now. These pockets of right now are perfect moments. It's not about never being disturbed again, but about ordinary moments lived in extraordinary ways.

☆ focusing meditation

You might think of Mindfulness Meditation as a sort of floodlight awareness: you simply allow things to arise and observe this stream of awareness without an agenda. One of the eight limbs of Hatha yoga, *dharana*, is about

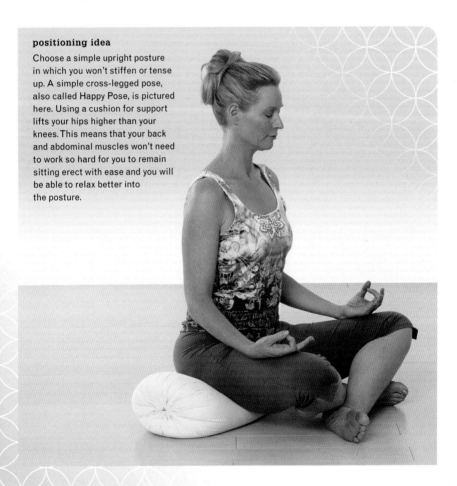

positioning idea

Choose a simple upright posture in which you won't stiffen or tense up. A simple cross-legged pose, also called Happy Pose, is pictured here. Using a cushion for support lifts your hips higher than your knees. This means that your back and abdominal muscles won't need to work so hard for you to remain sitting erect with ease and you will be able to relax better into the posture.

developing the ability to focus intently on a single point. Shining a light on this point is like a spotlight awareness, which paves the way for the next step – the following limb of Hatha yoga – which is meditation (*dhyana*).

1. Choose your most comfortable upright position. Close your eyes and settle in. Use relaxed belly-breathing. Notice how when you inhale, your abdomen expands first, followed by your chest as the air is drawn into your lungs. But don't try too hard; simply allow what is there to be there.

2. When you give your busy mind this little job to do, you will zone into the present moment and stress tends to fall away. Inhale and apply a mental count of one to that inhalation. Exhale and again count one. Inhale and mentally count two. Exhale and think two. Inhale and mentally say three. Exhale three. Inhale four. Exhale four. On your next inhalation, return to one, so that your next sequence repeats in exactly the same way: One and one. Two and two. Three and three. Four and four. Then return to one again.

3. Continue for eight full rounds. Then cease the counting, but continue resting your full attention on the simple act of breathing in and out. Most likely your mind will be quieter, as you have now trained it just to sit on the breath, as lightly as a butterfly will sit on a flower. You are now meditating on your breath. Stay as long as you wish: ten or 20 minutes is good (set a timer beforehand, if you wish). If you have time, it's good to resist that first and second urge to move out of this practice. Take the urge to move as an invitation to go deeper.

gratitude meditation

This practice reminds us that happiness comes from within, and it is a state of mind. It shifts us from negativity into abundance and prosperity. Gratitude reduces fear, helps us smile during the hard times and builds our relationships, as it eliminates resentment and reduces recrimination. Although there is sadness

positioning idea

From a high kneeling position, separate your feet and then sit down between them, in a seated Hero Pose. Use a prop such as a folded blanket or yoga block under the buttocks, if you wish. Rest your hands on your thighs.

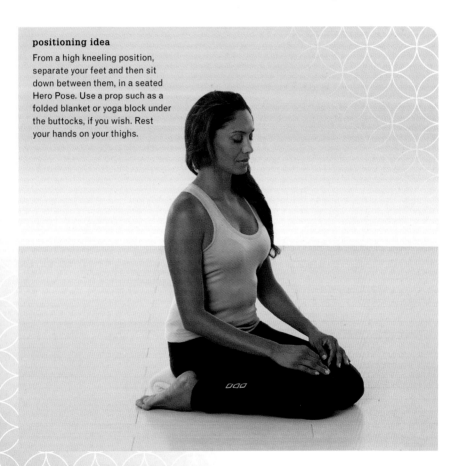

and suffering in the world, it's not disloyal to embrace the happiness we have. This practice helps us appreciate the true value of simple things. When we open to gratitude, we open to joy. Once we open to joy, we can be happy for ourselves and for others. Go forth and live in an attitude of gratitude.

1. Sit and centre yourself. Imagine that you have just tasted your favourite food. There's an appreciative sound that goes with that. Let the sound of *mmmmmmm* arise spontaneously. Over your next few breaths, inhale quietly, then exhale; as you exhale, make the nice, slow *mmmmmmm* sound aloud. Over the following breaths, let the sound quieten a little. Even when it is barely audible, observe how it still resonates through your body.

2. Now bring to mind the simple things that you have and love. It might be the nature around you, a sunny day or a good laugh.

3. Consider the special people in your life. Consider those who care for you, and those who cared for you in the past. Bring to mind the previous generations who came before you. Trusted friends. Your community.

4. Consider the health, well-being and safe harbour you have been given. Bring to mind with gratitude the teachings you have received. Just let your stream of consciousness flow. What you focus your mind on will naturally tend to expand. How positive it is to bring to mind all these wonderful blessings.

5. Let go of sounding your sounds of gratitude. Stay sitting and let the vibrations of the sound continue to resonate. Once the vibrations dissipate, let your breath be your focal point. Observe any effects of doing this practice. Then open your eyes.

☆ loving-kindness meditation

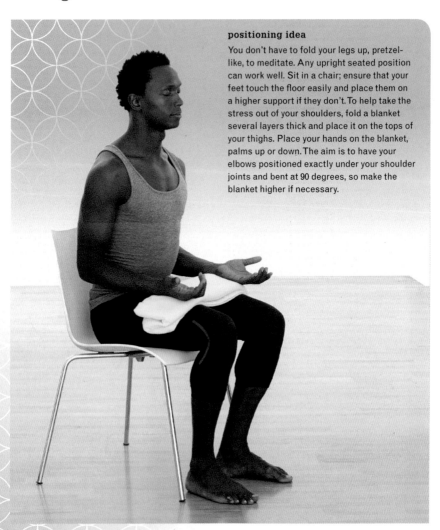

positioning idea

You don't have to fold your legs up, pretzel-like, to meditate. Any upright seated position can work well. Sit in a chair; ensure that your feet touch the floor easily and place them on a higher support if they don't. To help take the stress out of your shoulders, fold a blanket several layers thick and place it on the tops of your thighs. Place your hands on the blanket, palms up or down. The aim is to have your elbows positioned exactly under your shoulder joints and bent at 90 degrees, so make the blanket higher if necessary.

There are many variations of this Loving-Kindness Meditation, and I believe each is of great value in our modern world. I have included a version that uses the breath as a really nice anchor. A good intention to start off with is to vow to open to this practice, for the benefit of all beings.

1. Sit comfortably upright. Close your eyes. Check that you are settled, and take time in the beginning to get rid of any last fidgets.

2. Start to observe your breath. Choose the most obvious place in your body for you to notice the breath.

3. Start to count your breaths. Every third time you breathe, mentally say to yourself, "May my body and mind be at ease."

4. Every fourth breath, mentally repeat the phrase, "May all beings be at ease in body and mind."

5. Continue this practice for five minutes, or much longer if you have time. Before you finish, notice how you are feeling. This practice expands your heart and allows you to feel connected by the swirling energy of love and goodwill to your family, community and beyond.

ancient wisdom for modern life: how can we avoid suffering?

HEYAM DUKHAM ANAGATAM
हेयं दुखं अनगतं
Yoga Sutras II:17

This *sutra* literally translates as "to prevent suffering which has not yet arrived". It tells us that while we can't change our past, we do have some potential to change the future, by whatever action we consciously choose in the present. Importantly, it reminds us that we must act now, to anticipate and avoid undesirable future consequences.

This is incredibly empowering to take on board: right now, in this present moment, is the only time you can influence what comes next. In addition, only if your mind is in a state of clarity will your thought-processes initiate action that will not leave any residue. Any residue will manifest as *dukham*, or suffering.

Naturally, we cannot achieve this state of perfect action overnight, or without effort. But most (or all) of us would prefer to reduce the potential for future suffering. Start with something simple that is not too challenging. Set a goal and check your progress in a short span of time, such as a week.

This is another area where we are struck by an interesting paradox: we are already perfect as we are. Yet, as a human being, being perfect in that imperfection is again very apparent. There is no one human who does not act imperfectly at least occasionally, so if your ideal is to live a life completely free from suffering, you will be setting yourself an impossible goal. With this in mind, it's useful to understand how you can practically reduce at least the frequency, if not the intensity, of your suffering that is yet to come.

When considering the suffering of the future, you need to determine a couple of things. The first is to figure out which scenarios are merely an invention of your mind – those things that you worry about, but which will probably never happen. Don't let yourself be tormented by any of those unlikely future scenarios.

On the other hand, you do need to consider carefully the likely outcomes of your current actions. This *sutra* reminds us to act now, in order to avoid pain in the future. It's the original concept of the adage "an ounce of prevention is better than cure". It's not rocket science – if you always do what you always do, you're always going to get what you always get. So this *sutra* reminds us to be both responsible and responsive.

Using this *sutra* can guide you in making choices that better serve you, such as what you choose to eat, the work you choose to do and how you do it. It is helpful when examining how you choose to exercise, and even when you need to back off from doing certain things that you might usually think of as healthy – such as doing weight-bearing yoga poses when your wrist is sore.

This *sutra* helps you in your relationships with the people around you that you know and love, and with those far away whom you will never even meet or really know about. It encompasses the rest of the world, too. Act consciously and with integrity, as this *sutra* guides your actions concerning the environment. Be thoughtful about what you buy, cut down on over-consumption, and recycle. Make decisions based on more than short-term security or economic goals.

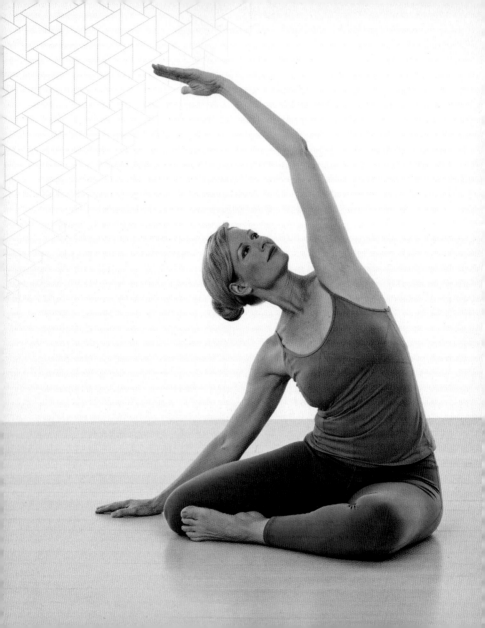

19

PUTTING IT ALL TOGETHER

Five practices

Here are five themed flows to kick-start your practice. These sequences will all offer you a nicely balanced practice. It is important to always factor in feedback from your body as you practice. At some point, you will feel ready to get creative and form your own sequences. As you do so, keep in mind that your body doesn't speak English, Spanish or Japanese. It has its own special language – the language of sensation. So be sure to attune yourself to the sensations of your body as you practice. Gather feedback from it during and after each pose. This "listening" to your body will guide you in selecting the next posture. That might be moving from a more active posture to a softer, soothing one. Perhaps it will be selecting a posture along the same path – moving from, say, a gentle forward bend to a deeper forward fold. Or maybe your body will ask for a pose that opposes the previous posture to help it balance out, such as taking a restful child's pose after an active inversion, or following a backbend with a twist. As you listen to the sensations of your body and respond to them, your yoga practice becomes truly yours. And it will feel like a pleasant, helpful and open conversation between good friends. Enjoy!

1. Power flow

Use the Three-Legged Dog between each of the standing postures and
between each side of the standing postures. For example, when you first come
into Exultant Warrior Flow, you'll take your left leg up and then lunge it forward.
Return to Classic Downward-Facing Dog Pose after that side, then take your

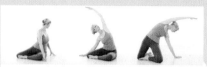

Spine Mobilizer (page 50)

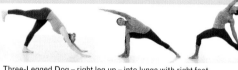

Strengthening Sun Salutation (page 76) x 3–6

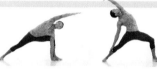

Exultant Warrior Flow (page 98)

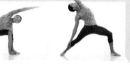

Three-Legged Dog – right leg up – into lunge with right foot
forward – Exultant Warrior Flow on right side

Three-Legged Dog – into lunge

Shoulder-Releasing Eagle (page 116)

Open Squat Twist (page 178)

East–West Flow (page 48)

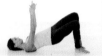

Dancing Bridge (page 202)

Plough-Pose Lifts (page 208)

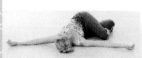

Reclining Eagle Twist (page 226)

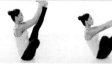

Half-Lotus Balance (page 166)

right leg up to lunge it forward for the second side of your Warrior. Set your holds in the static poses to suit you; three to five breaths is good. Use the Ocean Breath (see page 332) throughout this sequence, until you get to the relaxation and meditation at the end.

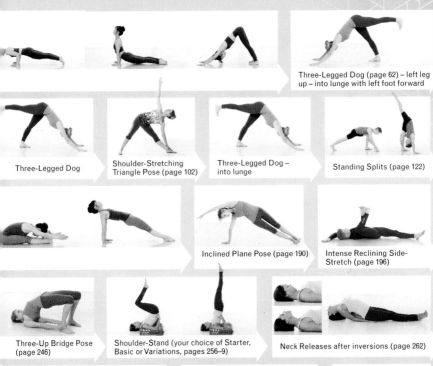

Three-Legged Dog (page 62) – left leg up – into lunge with left foot forward

Three-Legged Dog

Shoulder-Stretching Triangle Pose (page 102)

Three-Legged Dog – into lunge

Standing Splits (page 122)

Inclined Plane Pose (page 190)

Intense Reclining Side-Stretch (page 196)

Three-Up Bridge Pose (page 246)

Shoulder-Stand (your choice of Starter, Basic or Variations, pages 256–9)

Neck Releases after inversions (page 262)

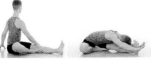

Head-Beyond-the-Knee Pose (page 160)

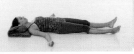

Peaceful Mind Relaxation (page 352)

Mindfulness Meditation (page 366)

2. Supple and strong flow

Here you can pepper your Sun Salutes with your standing postures. Do one complete round of the Sun Salute and then, each time you come into the Classic Downward-Facing Dog Pose after the Cobra, take the Dog-Pose Split and lunge the raised foot forward, so that you are ready for your standing posture.

START

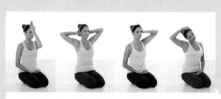

Seated Neck Stretch and Strengthen (page 134)

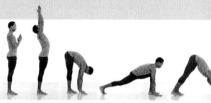

Easy Sun Salute (page 72)

Dog-Pose Split – lunge foot forward

Bound Side-Angle Stretch

Dog-Pose Split – lunge foot forward

Revolved Half-Moon Flow (page 110)

Dog Pose Spl each side

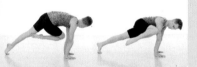

Core-Activating Plank Flow (page 212)

Threaded Needle (page 180)

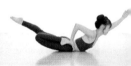

Half-Frog, Half-Locust (page 236)

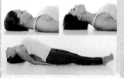

Neck Releases after Inversions (page 262)

Three-Step Reclining Twist (page 170)

Once you have completed the first side, come to standing again.
Complete the other half of your Sun Salute, ready to lunge the second
leg forward, for side two of the standing posture. Use the Ocean Breath
(see page 332) through the active part of the sequence.

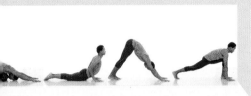

Dog-Pose Split (page 63)
– lunge foot forward

Bound Side-Angle
Stretch (page 104)

Dancer's Bow (page 124)

Big-Toe Balance
(page 126)

Crow to Plank Jump-Backs (page 148)

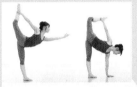
Sage Pose with Neck Releases (page 176)

Hip-Opening Heron Pose
(page 164)

Headstand
(pages 264–71)

Tibetan Alternate-Nostril Breathing (page 338)

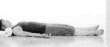
Serenity Relaxation
(page 348)

Gratitude Meditation
(page 370)

SUPPLE AND STRONG FLOW

3. Energy and balance

Use the Ocean Breath (see page 332) throughout this sequence, as it will help you feel strong, long and limber.

(see page 332)

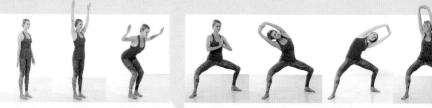

Chair-Pose Flow (page 88)

Dragon Flow (page 46)

Shoulder-Releasing Eagle (page 116)

Pyramid Prayer (page 140)

Deep Forward Bend at the Wall (page 152)

Twisted Pigeon (page 182)

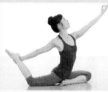

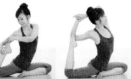

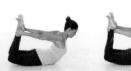

Pigeon Crescent Pose (page 242)

Bow Pose Three Ways (page 238)

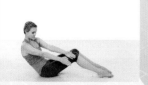

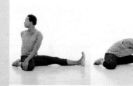

Seated Yogic Roll-Downs (continued)

Seated Rotated Gate (page 162)

Forearm Balance (page 276)

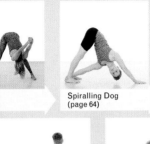

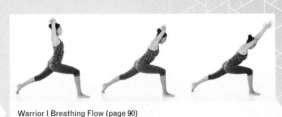

Spiralling Dog
(page 64)

Warrior I Breathing Flow (page 90)

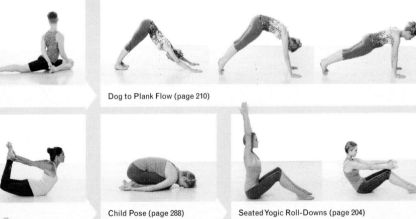

Dog to Plank Flow (page 210)

Child Pose (page 288)

Seated Yogic Roll-Downs (page 204)

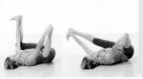

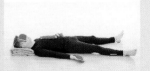

Heavenly Happy-Baby Pose
(page 158)

Energy-Balancing Relaxation
(page 350)

Focusing Meditation
(page 368)

4. Stretch and restore

You'll feel your body open and warm
with the active part of the practice, and
then enjoy the rewards of the restorative
postures to finish. Use the Ocean Breath
(page 332) through the active practices.

START

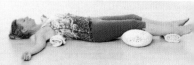

Backbend Ripple (page 290), using
Rectangular Breath (page 334)

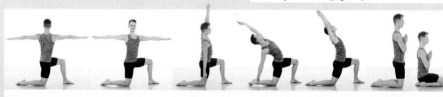

Salute to the Moon (continued)

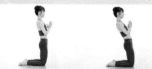

Seaweed Sway

Sugar-Cane Goddess
Pose (page 120)

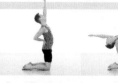

Shoulder-Releasing Forward Fold (page 108)

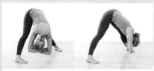

Prayer Sweeps (page 206)

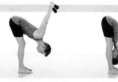

Camel Flow (page 244)

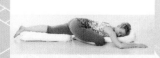

Resting Pigeon (page 294)

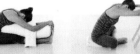

Restorative Forward Bends (page 296)

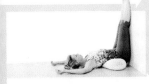

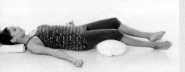

Salute to the Moon (page 80)

Double-Twist Dog Pose (page 65)

Seaweed Sway (page 106)

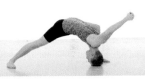

Bowing Side-Angle Pose (page 100)

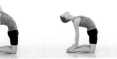

Kinky Cobbler's Pose (page 154)

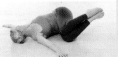

Yogic Compass (page 200)

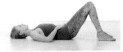

Corkscrew Twist (page 172)

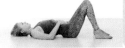

Blissful Banana (page 286)

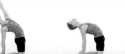

Restorative Inversion (page 298)

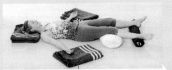

Floating Relaxation (page 354)

Loving-Kindness Meditation (page 372)

5. Clear and calm

This practice helps to slow and clear the mind, and mixes tension-releasing active yang postures with slow, focusing yin postures.

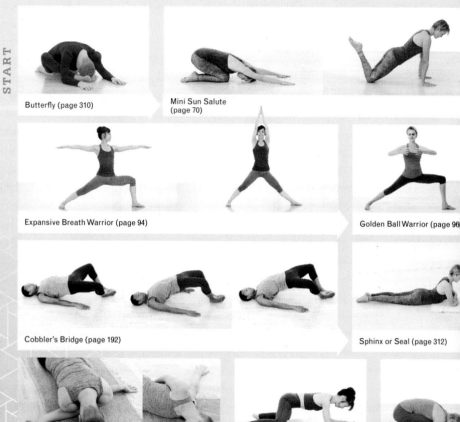

Butterfly (page 310)

Mini Sun Salute (page 70)

Expansive Breath Warrior (page 94)

Golden Ball Warrior (page 96)

Cobbler's Bridge (page 192)

Sphinx or Seal (page 312)

Yin Shoulder Stretches (page 322)

Yin Frog (page 324)

Child Pose (page 288)

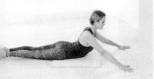

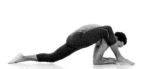

Yin Dragon Lunge (page 320)

Slinky Shoulders,
Gleeful Glutes (page 142)

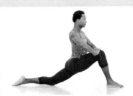

Tension-Releasing Forward Fold
(page 156)

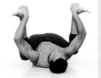

Yin Happy Baby (page 318)

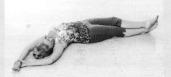

Banana Pose (page 194)

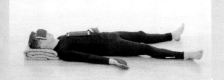

Energy-Balancing Relaxation (page 350)

Mindfulness
Meditation (page 366)

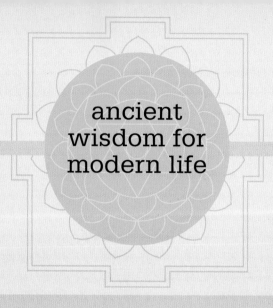

ancient wisdom for modern life

This traditional Indian greeting is often used to close a yoga class. It comes from two words: *Namas*, which means "bowing"; and *te*, meaning "to you". Most concisely it means "I bow down to you." But it runs deeper than that. *Namaste* means there is a special flame or divinity within each of us. And in salutation we acknowledge this spirit and bow down to honour the unique spirits in each other.

Its essence can be expanded out to the profound and bonding understanding that we are all of the same divine consciousness:

I honour the place in you where the entire universe resides.

I honour the place of light, love, truth, beauty and peace within you because it is also within me.

When you are in that place in you, and I am in that place in me, we are one.

NAMASTE नमस्ते

नमस्ते

Thank you for picking up this
book, and best wishes for
your journey onward.

Namaste,

Christina

glossary

agni In ayurvedic medicine, *agni* is the digestive fire, which, if it is healthy, helps us "digest" not only food but life experiences and impressions.

anterior An anatomical term referring to the front of the body.

asanas Literally meaning seat in Sanskrit, *asana* is the word used for a yoga posture.

Astanga yoga A flowing style of yoga taught by Pattabhi Jois in Mysore, India, which became popular in the West in the 1990s.

bandha In Sanskrit, *bandha* means lock. The three most commonly used energetic locks in Hatha yoga are those created by contractions around the pelvic floor, the lower abdomen and at the throat.

chi A Chinese word meaning life force or energy. It is similar to *prana* in Sanskrit.

cervical spine The seven neck vertebrae at the top of the vertebral column.

contraindicated A movement or treatment that is inadvisable under certain situations or conditions.

core muscles The muscles of the core include the abdominal muscles, pelvic floor muscles, some back muscles and the diaphragm muscle.

core-strengthening A practice that tones the core muscles.

counterpose A posture that opposes a preceeding posture to balance out its effects. For example, a forward bend or a twist will counterpose a backbend.

facet joints Also called zygapophyseal joints, these are small joints that sit between the articular processes of two adjacent vertebrae.

flow-state/flow-zone A mental state of operation in which a person performing an activity is fully immersed in feelings of energized focus and enjoyment in the activity.

free-balance The ability to bear full weight on the arms or hands without the use of any supporting structure.

gluteal muscles The buttocks each contain three muscles: the gluteus maximus, gluteus medius and gluteus minimus.

gunas One of the three qualities of nature, which are passion (*rajas*), dullness or inertia (*tamas*), and goodness or purity (*sattva*).

Hatha yoga Most modern styles of yoga are Hatha yoga, encompassing the eight limbs described on pages 12–13 and including the yoga postures.

heart centre The area at the centre of the chest corresponds to the heart chakra, an energy centre relating to compassion and unconditional love.

iliotibial band Also known as the IT band, this is a thick band of fascia that runs from the pelvis down the outer thigh to just below the knee.

Iyengar yoga Developed by BKS Iyengar, this style of Hatha yoga is characterized by long holds in the postures and the use of props such as belts, bolsters and bricks.

Kaivalya The absolute true state of consciousness, which is beyond the constraints of birth, existence and destruction.

karma yoga The "yoga of action", this is the path of selfless service to achieve the goal of enlightenment.

"limbs" of Hatha yoga The eight limbs are the *Yamas*, *Niyamas*, *Asana*, *Pranayama* (restraint of the breath), *Pratyahara* (withdrawl of the senses), *Dharana* (concentration), *Dhyana* (meditation) and *Samadhi* (bliss state).

lumbar spine The five vertebrae of the lower back, which are positioned above the sacral bone and below the thoracic vertebrae.

meridian (system) Channels that allow the movement of

subtle energies (such as *chi* or *prana*) in the body.

mindfulness Being aware of the present moment. Achieving this state, and calmly accepting one's feelings, thoughts and sensations, is highly therapeutic.

mudra A symbolic gesture, often made using the hands. *Mudras* are used to provide an energetic shift during yoga practices of asana, breathing and meditation

neuroplasticity The process in which the pathways of your brain are reorganized in response to environmental and behavioural changes.

niyama Practices of self-discipline and spiritual observances. The five *niyamas* are cleanlines, contentment, discipline, self-study and surrender to the divine.

paraspinal muscles The muscles next to the spine that support the movements of the vertebral column.

pelvic floor The muscles that span the bottom of the pelvis, forming the base of the abdomen.

posterior An anatomical term that refers to the back of the body.

prana A Sanskrit word for life-giving force. *Prana* also means breath.

pranayama The control of the breath. There are many

pranayama (breathing) practices in Hatha yoga.

puruśa The eternal and true Self. Pure consciousness, unaffected by external events.

prakriti Everything in the universe that is subject to change: all matter and also our thoughts, memories and desires.

quadriceps muscles The large muscle at the front of the thigh, which acts to extend (straighten) the leg.

sacroiliac joint The joint at the back of the pelvis, between the sacrum and the ilium bones

sacrum The triangular bone at the base of the lower back. This broad bony plate is made up of five fused vertebrae.

Samadhi A state of meditative consciousness, or trance-like absorption. This highest stage of meditation is one of the limbs of Hatha yoga.

Samkhya One of six orthodox schools of Hindu philosophy.

samskara Impressions, ideas or mental imprints that make up our psychological conditioning.

the Self The pure and divine within us, also referred to as the true Self. The small-s self, created by the ego, gives a false sense of self.

self-realization
Understanding the Self as pure awareness and therefore the

fulfillment of one's potential. A state free of ego.

sitting bones The two bony bumps upon which we usually place our weight while sitting, the technical term for which is the ischial tuberosity.

solar plexus An energy centre or *chakra* located just above the navel.

sutra A precept summarizing a teaching. The *Yoga Sutras* is an ancient text, written by Patanjali, that codified yoga.

synovial capsule A cavity formed by the smooth cartilage that covers the bones of a joint.

synovial fluid A viscous fluid found in the cavities of synovial joints, which reduces friction between the cartilage of the joints during movement.

thoracic spine/vertebrae
The section of the vertebral column in the upper and middle region of the back, below the neck. The thoracic spine has 12 vertebrae.

Veda A large collection of texts forming the earliest body of Indian sacred writings.

Vedanta One of six orthodox schools of Hindu philosophy.

yama Practices of ethical standards. The five *yamas* are: non-violence, truthfulness, non-stealing, sexual continence and non-covetousness.

GLOSSARY

index

INDEX

acknowledgements

Thank you, Jerry, for your cheerful support – you insist you are soulless, yet your soulful and steady natural yogi state supports me more than you can know. To my shiny-eyed, joyful Safia, thanks for her patience with Mummy's last 30 pages of the book. You are my mirror, who shines a light on my life, and I love you more than words can ever express. And to my precious bundle of cuddly love, Asha, your occasional 4am alarm bell helped this book to get written. At any time of the day or night, you will always make my heart swell.

Good childcare can make all the difference to a mum. Every class I teach is a little creation in itself, and this book was a slightly more time-consuming one. My heartfelt thanks to Madeleine Geist, Jennifer Kollmann and Yutika U-Pongthong (Noona), who allowed me some time away from putting Vegemite on toast and freed me up to create. Maddie was in our lives as I opened Transform, my latest yoga studio, when my youngest daughter was not quite two. Jenny was there with her wonderful supportive energy as the business grew enough to enable me to even consider this endeavour. And Noona took such good care of my little ones, and us, during the writing of this book.

Thanks to all those around the world who bought the original classic, The Yoga Bible, and therefore made the creation of this book possible.

To all my students: you make it possible for me to do what I love, and even to make a living from it. How lucky am I?!

Thanks to Kristen Blackwell, Em Cruikshank and Rosemary Bekker, for checking that I actually wrote in English, not "yoga". Kristen knew me before I knew her, from having owned a copy of The Yoga Bible in America, and then, by my good fortune, turned out to be an excellent next-door neighbour in Sydney. Rosie, your weekly check-ins over chai tea are cherished. Em sets an auspicious vibe in her gorgeous yin classes.

Lunches with fellow writers Mischa Telford and Jayne Tancred offered clarity on the curvy pathway to planning out this book, and their wise words dissolved a couple of hurdles on the path forward. Thank you, Mischa, for your excellent yoga history and philosophy support. I always love your briliant analogies and fascinating observations.

Thanks to Louise and Richard G for their writing space with a view. Thanks to our yogi and yogini models Emi Takahashi Tull, Paul Anderson, Daniel Breakwell (dbreakyoga.com), Anne Thomson (http://annethomson314.wixsite.com/anne-thomson-yoga), Meera Anderson (manifestingdestiny.com.au) and Richard James Allen (physicaltv.com.au) for making the shoot flow. Thank you to the wonderful Melanie DeSylva for beautiful hair and the fabulous Wendy Smith and Kristy and Andrew Pownell for wardrobe support.

In any life – ancient or modern – there is suffering. Yet in its way, sadness is life-affirming. To my niece Laura Acton, a blossom, who we all achingly miss: you would just have been turning 21 now. Your presence lives with us every day and you remind me what is important in life.